The Complete Guide to
Alternative Cancer Therapies

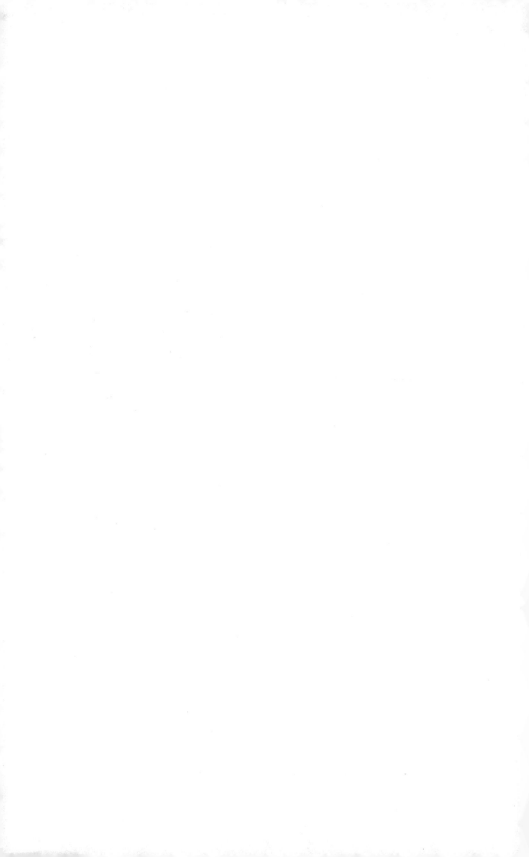

The Complete Guide to Alternative Cancer Therapies

*What You Need to Know
to Make an Informed Choice*

Ron Falcone

A CITADEL PRESS BOOK
Published by Carol Publishing Group

A Citadel Press Book
Published by Carol Publishing Group
Citadel Press is a registered trademark of Carol Communications, Inc.
Editorial Offices: 600 Madison Avenue, New York, N.Y. 10022
Sales and Distribution Offices: 120 Enterprise Avenue, Secaucus, N.J. 07094
In Canada: Canadian Manda Group, P.O. Box 920, Station U, Toronto, Ontario   M8Z 5P9
Queries regarding rights and permissions should be addressed to Carol Publishing Group,
600 Madison Avenue, New York, N.Y. 10022
Carol Publishing Group books are available at special discounts for bulk purchases, sales
promotions, fund raising, or educational purposes. Special editions can be created to
specifications. For details, contact Special Sales Department, Carol Publishing Group,
120 Enterprise Avenue, Secaucus, N.J. 07094

The author and publisher do not accept responsibility for any decisions made by the reader
regarding health care choices. The purpose of this book is solely to provide information and
serve as a reference guide and is not meant to be interpreted or construed as advice on
cancer treatment. Persons who wish to seek alternative cancer treatment should consult an
experienced health care professional and, preferably, one who is experienced in holistic,
alternative modes of therapy.

Manufactured in the United States of America

10 9 8 7 6 5 4 3 2 1

Library of Congress Cataloging-in-Publication Data

Falcone, Ron.
    The complete guide to alternative cancer therapies: what you need
to know to make an informed choice / by Ron Falcone.
        p. cm.
    "A Citadel Press book."
    ISBN 0–8065–1553–8 (pbk.)
    1. Cancer—Alternative treatment.   I. Title.
RC271.A62F35   1994
616.99'406—dc20
                                                        94–17473
                                                          CIP

To all cancer patients, their families, and those dedicated to the conquest of cancer in spite of tremendous adversity.

Contents

Acknowledgments

I would like to thank the following people for their generosity, valuable advice, and encouragement:

Alan Cantwell M.D., for his expertise, guidance, enlightenment and compassion; Alva H. Johnson PhD, for his time, consideration and for helping to shed light on an important piece of the cancer puzzle; the late Virginia Livingston M.D. for kindly sharing her published data and remarkable expertise; Kenneth Forror M.D. of the Livingston Clinic for his advice and time; Burton Waisbren M.D., for reading a portion of the manuscript and for his suggestions; Joseph Gold M.D. for his data and published studies; Wolfram W. Kuhnau M.D. for his enthusiastic answers to many questions.

Thanks also to: Michael Culbert, President of the Committee for Freedom of Choice in Medicine, for shedding important light on a controversial subject and for sending very helpful materials; Lee Trombetta of the Burzynski Research Institute for her prompt and courteous reply in sending valuable information; Carol Case R.N. and Christy Thomsen of the National Cancer Institute for their informative letters and generous forwarding of data; the American Cancer Society for generously supplying me with many pages of information; Lorraine Rosenthal of the Cancer Control Society for helping to keep me informed over the years; the friendly staff of the Bridgeport, Connecticut Public Library (Burroughs Branch) for helping me in more ways than they know; the staff of the Yale University School of Medicine library for kindly allowing me unlimited use of their remarkable archives.

I'd like to extend a special thanks to Steven Schragis, my publisher at Carol Publishing Group, for having faith in this project early on and to Denise O'Sullivan, my editor, for her patience, valuable suggestions and support in the revision and completion of the manuscript.

Finally, to my wife Anne for all she has done to keep this book alive and for having to put up with me while it was being written.

Preface

For all their hazards and expense, the three mainstays of orthodox cancer treatment—radiation, surgery, and chemotherapy—have not appreciably altered the epidemic of cancer that continues to claim millions of lives every year.

Certainly, one of the most formidable conceptual problems with current treatments is that they do not attack the underlying causes of cancer; if cancer does have a genetic, viral, or immunological basis, then poisoning, cutting, or irradiating will not reverse those factors and may even provoke the cancer process.

In recent years, a good deal of research has focused on the role that immunity plays in tumor causation. Once considered theoretical, the immunity factor is being viewed with increasing significance and few scientists would totally dispute its relationship to cancer. Several studies have shown, for example, that immunity suppressing drugs used in organ transplants increase the risk of lymphomas, leukemias, and other types of cancer in humans (1, 2). Since cancer treatments interfere with the production of antibodies and other disease-fighting cells, critics have long questioned the logic and validity of their use.

Undoubtedly, the appeal of unorthodox cancer therapies has been due, in large part, to their "body-friendly" nature. Indeed, a number of people are choosing them if for no other reason than to avoid treatments seen as harmful and toxic. But there is always a danger that natural, "holistic" treatments are not medically sound and will be chosen in place of standard procedures which have been shown to cure. It is here that choices must be weighed by the most careful and sensible review of all available information. That some toxic therapies do, in fact, work should preclude a universal rejection of them. But the public, in its increasing skepticism, has sent a strong signal to the medical community that there *has to be* a better way to help resolve the suffering millions of human beings must endure in the struggle to combat cancer.

The Complete Guide to
Alternative Cancer Therapies

Introduction

National cancer agencies in the United States maintain a vigorous stance against most alternative cancer therapies. All the while, they continue to espouse chemotherapy, surgery, and radiation as the only scientifically "proven" mainstays of treatment. In recent years, however, a growing consensus among critics, the public, and even cancer practitioners has forced all but the staunchest defenders of conventional medicine to admit one inescapable fact: convincing evidence shows that the officially approved treatments cure only a small percentage of those with the disease and in most cases do not improve the quality of life of those being treated.

In some instances, scientific documentation has shown that cancer patients may actually worsen and even develop new tumors as a direct result of medical treatment.

Such depressing statistics are not new and have worried government leaders for decades. As early as 1971, President Richard Nixon signed into law the National Cancer Act heralding official "war" on the disease. Mustering the unprecedented support of Congress and enlisting the best scientific talent, Nixon promised a cure by 1976—the year of the American bicentennial.

The primary focus of research would be to unravel a cancer-virus link in humans. Scientists were confident that once this link was established, the development of effective vaccines would help solve the cancer riddle.[1] A massive effort was thus under way, fueled by billions of tax dollars and a public confident in the unquestioned legacy of its medical technology.

The bicentennial came and went, and still no cure was in sight. By 1979, enthusiasm over the virus link began to sour, and this prompted

National Cancer Institute (NCI) chief Dr. Arthur Upton to revise earlier projections and reluctantly admit that "it would be wrong to expect a cure soon."[2] Two years later, NCI investigators finally concluded that viruses only played a minor role in cancer causation and even *that* link was tenuous.[3] Besides the virus setback, national cancer agencies were grappling with yet another dilemma. Despite their best efforts at containing and preventing the spread of cancer within the patient via programs of prevention and early diagnosis, the disease continued growing at an alarming rate, becoming the second leading cause of death among Americans by the 1980s.[4]

Seemingly indifferent to this growing body of facts, leading cancer experts optimistically stated that because "progress is so encouraging"[5] and "milestones" are being achieved against cancer,[6] it was only a matter of time before a "cure" would be discovered. But in 1986, this optimism was dealt a staggering blow when a report in the *New England Journal of Medicine* concluded that the war on cancer was, in fact, a failure.[7] An equally scathing indictment was issued by a high-level federal advisory board who found that the rate of successfully cured cancer patients had hardly improved in thirty years for most major types of the disease.[8] By 1988, it had become clear that most of the gains made against cancer occurred primarily between 1960 and 1974; since then, five-year survival rates have only increased less than *1 percent*.[9]

Three decades after President Nixon's declaration, the cancer puzzle remains as formidable and elusive as ever. And despite an estimated 1 trillion dollars having been spent on research,[10] the death toll from the disease continues to climb. Nonetheless, the American Cancer Society (ACS) and other national agencies continue to tell the public that cancer—if diagnosed early—could be cured in half of all cases.[11] Further, official progress reports show cancer patients to be living longer than at any other time in history. But these reports may be creating a false sense of progress due to biases in the way statistics are tabulated.

For example, cancer patients may seem to live longer today due to earlier diagnosis of their disease (made possible via advanced technologies) and *not* because of better treatment. According to a federal advisory board, this fact alone "virtually guarantees" five-year survival (the time frame which, in the absence of any disease recurrence, usually constitutes a "cure") even if people are not actually cured in the long term.[12] In addition, a Harvard University disease expert has called improved cancer survival a "statistical artifact" created by the declining incidence of deadly cancers that were once common.[13]

In other facets of cancer reporting, statistics appear to be favorably influenced by the selective manipulation of data. For example, 600,000 cases of skin cancer and 100,000 cases of other localized cancers are reported each year in the United States and yet these are *excluded* from the national statistics.[14] In a candid interview, Irving Rimer, a former vice president of information at the ACS explained that omitting such a vast number of cancers from the total annual cases undoubtedly creates the "appearance" of declining cancer rates.[15] Indeed, the General Accounting Office confirmed, in a 1987 report, that the NCI's fact-gathering methods were biased, creating an "artificially inflated amount of true progress."[16]

True progress against cancer may also be exaggerated, oddly enough, by the official definition of "cure." For instance, if a recovering cancer patient relapses *after* the five-year cure deadline, the new diagnosis can theoretically count as a unique case while the original "cure" remains on the books.[17] This scenario may happen routinely and thus falsely inflate cure rates. But even when cures appear to be valid, the exact number of people actually benefiting from cancer treatment remains a subject of intense controversy.

By the ACS's own admission, only *40* percent of all Americans afflicted with cancer are actually cured—not half as is generally claimed.[18] The ACS explains this discrepancy by noting that if people with cancer did not die from other causes before finishing treatment, 50 percent *could* be cured.*[19] However, there is no precise way to measure just how many patients would benefit if allowed to finish a full course of treatment. The ACS's 50 percent claim is thus a best-case scenario and does not reflect real data.

Perhaps the most deceiving element of the "50 percent" claim is that it creates a false expectation of cure. The fact is, recovery rates for cancer are so variable that a median-line cure "average" for individuals is practically meaningless.

Depending on the type, location, and stage of cancer as well as a multiplicity of other factors, cure rates can range from 1 to better than 90 percent.[20]

---

*This artificially projected cure number is known as the "relative survival rate." The true rate of about 40 percent is called the "observed rate."

Figure 1
Five-Year Average* Cancer Survival Rates
(Percent) for Selected Sites, by Race

Site	**Relative Five-Year Survival Rates (Percent)	
	White	Black
All Sites	52	38
Oral Cavity and Pharynx	53	31
Esophagus	9	6
Stomach	16	18
Colon	57	48
Rectum	54	41
Liver	5	4
Pancreas	3	4
Larynx	69	52
Lung and Bronchus	13	11
Melanoma, Skin	81	65
Breast (Female)	78	64
Cervix	67	57
Corpus Uteri	84	55
Ovary	39	38
Prostate	75	62
Testis	92	92
Urinary Bladder	70	59
Kidney	53	51
Brain & Nervous System	24	32
Thyroid	94	96
Hodgkin's Disease	76	74
Non-Hodgkin's Lymphomas	51	45
Multiple Myeloma	26	28
Leukemia	36	29

*Average survival rates do not take into account the patient's status at time of diagnosis nor do they indicate the prognosis based on the particular stage or degree of illness one is diagnosed at. For example, while ovarian cancer has a 39 percent cure average (for white patients), more than half of all sufferers are actually diagnosed after the disease has spread, at which time "cure" rates drop to only 18 percent.

**Relative survival rates are not true percentages of cure since they are based on artificial projections (see also page 5, this chapter).

Source: American Cancer Society.

Consider that thyroid cancer—which accounts for about 1 percent of total malignancies in the U.S.—can be successfully treated about 90 percent of the time.[21] But carcinoma of the lung, which is the leading cancer killer among Americans, has only a 13 percent cure rate average.[22] And cancer of the pancreas—which claims 25,000 U.S. lives

Figure 2
Observed Three-year Survival Rates (Percent),
By Age, 1985 to 1988

Primary Site	Number of Cases	0–19	20–49	50–59	60–69	70–79	80 +	Total
Oral Cavity/Pharynx	3,464	78	72	60	55	48	40	56
Esophagus	1,048	—	—	10	13	10	—	11
Stomach	1,810	—	22	25	24	19	17	21
Colon	8,948	100	66	64	63	57	45	57
Rectum	4,129	—	66	65	63	56	43	58
Liver	516	43	18	5	6	4	4	8
Gallbladder	570	—	29	31	22	14	16	19
Pancreas	1,837	—	12	5	4	4	1	4
Larynx	1,647	—	77	73	67	59	44	66
Lung and Bronchus	14,629	—	19	20	18	13	7	16
Bone	309	69	81	73	45	63	—	69
Soft Tissue	749	76	58	70	60	61	47	61
Melanoma, Skin	4,101	91	76	85	80	75	58	76
Breast	14,627	—	85	85	85	80	65	82
Cervix	1,862	—	79	63	60	55	41	69
Corpus Uteri	2,209	—	93	87	81	74	49	79
Ovary	1,198	100	74	51	43	31	19	47
Other Female	429	—	90	64	69	60	47	64
Prostate	8,467	—	71	83	81	75	52	73
Testis	745	93	91	92	89	—	—	91
Urinary Bladder	3,695	83	87	81	72	61	44	65
Kidney	2,070	90	63	61	59	53	39	58
Eye	261	92	92	79	78	70	51	80
Central Nervous System	2,094	70	62	21	12	8	9	34
Thyroid Gland	1,020	100	98	92	76	61	35	89
Hodgkin's Disease	876	92	90	71	56	47	25	81
Non-Hodgkin's Lymphomas	2,854	70	60	64	54	41	24	50
Multiple Myeloma	939	—	67	43	37	34	25	37
Leukemia	2,144	62	41	40	29	25	15	35

Survival rates for groups of less than 10 patients are not reported.
Source: American Cancer Society.

annually—is still a virtual death sentence, killing more than 95 percent of its victims[23] (see Figure 1).

Further, the variability of cure within a certain age group can be tremendous. For instance, while cancers affecting the brain and nervous system are considered 70 percent treatable for patients under twenty years of age, the cure rate drops to a grim *12 percent* for people sixty years of age or older (see Figure 2).

Burdened with such gloomy reports and a growing crisis of credibility, officials have attempted to shift attention toward those advances in treatment that have been made. For example, in recent years much publicity has been given to the enormous progress being made against leukemia. There have been continued appeals for public donations and a barrage of highly emotive television commercials popularizing how we are "winning the war" against leukemia. But while survival rates for the most treatable forms of this disease have risen by as much as 67 percent, the highest average rate of cure for *all* forms of leukemia combined is only 36 percent.[24]

Disturbingly, the 36 percent leukemia cure rate is actually based on figures gathered for whites; blacks have only a 29 percent chance of recovering from the disease.[25] In fact, overall cure rates for blacks have not been included in government reports which proclaim the progress being made against cancer.[26] Why? According to the authors of the *NEJM* study, including the black rates with the general population would "depress the statistics" since blacks suffer from a higher incidence of untreatable cancers.[27]

Unable to deny the fact that cancer deaths in the United States continue to escalate despite aggressive medical intervention, experts insist that recovery rates *could* be better *if* only diagnoses were made early enough. But according to the NCI, such cancers as those of the lung, esophagus, liver, and pancreas remain largely incurable, *even* when diagnosis is performed at the earliest, most opportune time.[28] And while enormous strides have been made in computer technology, ultrasound, fiber optics, and the entire gamut of high-tech medical diagnostics, a growing body of clinical evidence suggests that for some cancers, cure rates have actually gotten *worse*.[29] In view of these disturbing facts, the actual value of the "approved" cancer therapies have come under bitter scrutiny in recent years.

Surgery, which is one of the first lines of defense against cancer, can traumatize people for life; in many cases, vital organs are removed and permanent and debilitating cosmetic and physical changes occur although the patient may be considered "cured."

Surgical excision is the oldest form of cancer treatment known, and it is now used for half of all cancer patients.[30] Often, the success of surgery is based on early and complete removal of malignant cells but, as already noted, this factor is not always present.[31]

A popular notion that has long been held is that surgery itself may spread cancer. In view of recent findings, this idea may not be so farfetched. One study has shown, for example, that of 1,532 lung-cancer patients who underwent complete surgical resection, 104 later developed brain cancers.[32] According to some clinicians, there may, in fact, be a causal relationship between surgery and malignancy; some evidence shows that surgery and related procedures such as needle biopsies may themselves spread malignant cells or other possible coagents that contribute to cancer.[33]

Even when cancer surgery does result in five-year cure rates, a major concern in the *quality* of life resulting from it. Consider, for example, radical surgery of the head and neck. In order to be effective, this type of surgery must often be extensive and mutilating and may necessitate removal of part or all of the lip, tongue, cheek, jawbones, and adjacent nerves.[34] Although many patients may suffer from these long-term complications, surgeons still recommend radical neck dissection as an "insurance" against the possible recurrence of cancer.[35]

Unfortunately, there does not appear to be a clear consensus on just when this drastic operation should be performed, and often the decision to do so depends on the personal beliefs and opinions of the surgeon and not on absolute, defined guidelines.[36] Such divergence of opinion may spell the difference between life-long debility and a reasonable quality of life. Indeed, the permanent disfigurement that often results from radical neck surgery can impact patients and lead to "profound" emotional reactions.[37] Depression, poor self-image and despondency are chronic and common complaints that may persist even though patients live past the five-year cure deadline.

Other traumatizing surgeries involving excision of limbs, reproductive organs, or parts of the nervous system might adequately remove tumors but leave patients infertile, impotent, and debilitated—sometimes for the rest of their lives. Patients who have had major gastrointestinal surgery, for instance, generally do not regain their capacity to eat and digest normal meals, have problems absorbing nutrients, and rarely regain normal strength. These patients often live in semi-invalid conditions with little hope for a long-term cure.[38]

Perhaps no one issue confounds people more than the extent to which cancer surgery should be performed. A case in point involves the radical mastectomy, which may involve entire removal of the breast, underlying chest muscles, and lymph nodes. For decades, radical breast surgery was the procedure of choice at the first sign of cancer. The operation is disfiguring and from a psychological standpoint, often devastating. Current evidence shows, however, that "breast-conserving surgery," which only removes the tumor and some surrounding tissue, is equally effective for early stage cancers.[39]

Despite the value of conservative, less-mutilating surgery, data shows that it is not always implemented even though it could be. Some studies have shown that older surgeons are more likely to resort to the radical procedure—their beliefs and practice methods more often determining their method of operation.[40] In addition, the patient's age, social background, selection of hospital and demographic region also weigh in the decision whether or not radical breast surgery will be performed. In this light, younger, better educated, and more affluent women are more likely to be treated with breast-conserving surgery.[41]

Considerable debate also centers around prostate cancer, the most commonly diagnosed malignancy afflicting men. Each year, 28,000 Americans die from this disease and the value of surgery has become equally controversial both in the extent to which it is necessary and in the quality of life it renders.

If diagnosed early, the chances of curing prostate cancer are good to excellent. Although the primary method of arresting the disease has been complete removal of the prostate, it is now believed that for some patients a "watchful waiting" approach may be better than surgery.[42] For other patients, removal of the prostate with all its attendant complications may be more effective.[43]

Total surgical removal of the prostate might indeed cure cancer, but permanent side effects include irreversible impotence, and for most men, this factor can hardly be considered an improvement in the quality of life. In more advanced forms of the disease, castration and the addition of female sex hormones is a prescribed course of treatment.[44] As in breast cancer, the rate of surgery on men with prostate cancer may vary according to regions of the United States.[45]

For many types of cancer, surgery is not usually performed as the sole procedure. In order to increase the odds of survival and to insure that malignant cells missed by the surgeon's knife do not proliferate, radiation treatments are often used adjunctively. For certain tumors difficult to access, radiation may be the only treatment of choice.

Radiation therapy was first pioneered in the 1920s, and ever since, there has been a good deal of publicity over its potential curative value. Unlike surgery, radiotherapy is not mutilating and can offer significant reversal of tumors or painful symptoms associated with cancer. In a number of cases, cures are achieved.

In recent years, improvements in diagnosis via computerized X-ray techniques such as CAT (computerized axial tomography) scans have made tumors easier to locate and target. Once identified, the delivery of a narrow beam of radiation to the affected cite hopefully eradicates malignant cells while incurring the least damage to healthy cells. In some cases, lasers are being tried on solid tumors such as those of the esophagus. Currently, more than 50 percent of all cancer patients receive radiation therapy at some point in their illness,[46] and the most commonly treated cancers are those of the breast, head and neck, larynx, bladder, and cervix.[47]

While the noninvasive treatment of cancer with radiation seems an ideal approach, radiotherapy still presents serious drawbacks that have not been solved. For example, radioactive materials are known to suppress or destroy key parts of the immune system, such as the disease-fighting B-cells.[48] Since many scientists now believe that immunity plays a crucial role in the prevention and even reversal of cancer, treatments that *weaken* the immune system may compromise overall health and the long-term prognosis of the patient.

Although the ultimate role that radiation plays on immunity is yet to be fully determined, a multitude of known side effects ranging from minor to disastrous have been documented and pose a formidable challenge to medical practitioners. Hair loss, severe irritation, nausea, and the general malaise associated with radiation sickness are more immediate symptoms of treatment. Sterility, premature aging, abnormal healing, bowel obstruction, and narrowing of the esophagus are other problems that may make themselves known over a period of time.[49]

Depending on where and to what extent therapy is carried out, radiation can cause problems that may affect patients for years or even a lifetime. For example, radiation used to treat brain tumors has been shown to result in a number of glandular abnormalities; in one study, almost all the treated patients developed endocrine problems, including hypothyroidism, growth hormone disturbances, lowered sexual hormones in men, and diminished or absent menstrual flow in women.[50] In another study, nearly half the patients undergoing therapy for Hodgkin's disease developed thyroid problems, eye disorders, and even thyroid cancers.[51] In children, irradiation of brain tumors has led to incomplete sexual development, retarded growth, and learning deficits.[52] Ironically, while some of these children were cured of their cancers, they suffered long-term consequences in adulthood that proved detrimental to their physical and psychic well-being.

Probably the most feared and paradoxical result of treatment is the onset of new cancers. It is well established that radiation—no matter how "safely" it is administered—causes abnormal changes in the chromosomes of healthy cells, predisposing them to malignancy. In some cases, people who are successfully "cured" experience the growth of secondary tumors years after therapy.

A tragic example involved the treatment of children with acute lymphoblastic leukemia (ALL). In the 1960s very few young patients survived this devastating illness, but today complete cure rates have approached 70 percent and, understandably, these achievements are often cited as the brightest stars in the war on cancer. However, ALL patients also have a twenty-two fold greater chance of developing brain tumors than do nontreated children.[53]

While the link between radiation therapy and cancer is certainly not a mystery and has been well charted, the *extent* of this link may still be underestimated. Investigators have found, for example, that when children were treated for a noncancerous condition with lower doses of radiation than normally used in cancer therapy[54] they still experienced a "significant increase" in the onset of brain tumors.[55] In adults, the correlation between secondary tumors and treatment is equally disquieting. For instance, a number of women who underwent radiation therapy for cancer in one breast later developed new tumors in the opposite breast.[56] A small number of women also experienced a greater risk of radiation-induced leukemia.[57]

Currently, the value of radiation therapy is being debated. While many clinicians believe the method is indispensable for some cancers and can offer significant palliation of symptoms, others question its true benefits. One leading critic is Harvard University professor John Cairns, whose scathing critique of the failed "war on cancer" predated the official negative report by the U.S. General Accounting Office. Cairns argues that radiation can never effectively cure "the majority of cancers"[58] because the dose required would prove lethal to most patients.[59]

While the ultimate value of surgery and radiation continue to provoke debate, chemotherapy has come under especially intense scrutiny in recent years. Considered by many the most toxic and dubious of the currently accepted treatments, cancer drugs are noted for often severe and sometimes fatal side effects (Figure 3).

Drugs must circulate in the bloodstream at or near peak levels of toxicity in order to work; ironically, it is the extent of this toxicity that often determines chemotherapy's success and, paradoxically, its potential destructiveness. That cancer drugs work at all lies in their ability to target faster growing cells (often a characteristic of cancer) as opposed to slower growing cells (usually a characteristic of healthy tissues).

Once fast-dividing cells are exposed to the drugs, a number of mechanisms take place that result in cell death. For example, some chemical agents interfere with DNA synthesis and disrupt the ability of cells to reproduce; other compounds prevent malignant cells from using certain nutrients needed for their survival. Unfortunately, healthy cells (for example, those making up the hair follicles, bone marrow, and stomach lining) grow rapidly and are themselves targeted and killed by cancer drugs; this lack of selectivity is chemotherapy's major drawback.

Damaged hair follicles often lead to baldness, a condition that usually reverses itself once therapy is discontinued. But damage to the gastrointestinal tract can result in a dangerous impairment of nutrient absorption. And suppression of blood-producing organs such as bone marrow can cause a weakened immunity, inability to fight infections, and even death.

A number of different drugs are now in use to treat specific forms of cancer (see Figure 4). One of the more commonly used chemotherapeutic agents is Methotrexate,[60] used against certain forms of lung, bone, head, neck, breast, and skin cancers. Oddly, the drug's mode of action is to interrupt the manufacture of folic acid, a B vitamin essential to life and a normally functioning body. Folic acid is also crucial in preventing chromosome damage—one of the very mechanisms by which cancer is believed to be caused in the first place. A lack of this essential vitamin may, in fact, play a key role in spurring the growth of new cancers.[61] Folic acid depletion is also associated with nervous system problems such as depression, and this condition can adversely affect immunity and, possibly, the prognosis of the patient.

Methotrexate presents a range of other adverse effects, including obstructive pulmonary disease, sterility, infertility, nausea, vomiting, baldness, and even death.[62] Due to these potentially grave complications, the drug's manufacturer issues the following warning to physicians:

Figure 3
Guide to Commonly Used Cancer Drugs

Drug	Indicated use	Major side effects
ANTIBIOTIC DERIVATIVES		
Adriamycin, Rubex (Doxorubicin hydrochloride)	Lymphomas, leukemia, bone sarcomas, breast, ovarian, bladder, thyroid, gastric, lung cancers; Hodgkin's disease	Heart failure, heart muscle destruction, bone marrow suppression, alopecia (baldness), severe nausea and vomiting, severe bleeding, colon tissue damage, allergic shock
Blenoxane (Bleomycin sulfate)	Palliative treatment of head, neck, cervical cancer. Also lymphomas, Hodgkin's disease and cancer of the sex organs	Pneumonia (10% frequency), occasionally pulmonary fibrosis, fever, chills, vomiting, anorexia, weight loss, severe allergic reactions
Cerubidine (Daunorubicin hydrochloride)	Acute leukemia	Severe cardiac toxicity, nausea, alopecia
Mithracin (Plicamycin)	Testicular cancer	Severe hemorrhage—possibly fatal; anorexia, nausea, vomiting, diarrhea
Mutamycin (Mitomycin)	Adjunctively used in the palliative treatment of stomach and pancreas cancer	Bone marrow suppression (sometimes permanent), occasional pulmonary toxicity, kidney failure, nausea, vomiting (infrequent)
ANTIMETABOLITES		
5-FU (Fluorouracil)	Palliative treatment of colorectal, breast, stomach, pancreatic cancer	Severe toxic reactions; hemorrhage, intractable vomiting, bone marrow suppression, alopecia, allergic reactions, death
Methotrexate	Acute leukemia, choriocarcinoma; cancers of the head, neck, bone, lung	Potentially serious lung disease, marked bone marrow suppression, severe diarrhea, fetal death, liver cirrhosis

Drug	Indications	Side Effects
Novantrone (Mitoxantrone hydrochloride)	Adult leukemias	Alopecia, nausea, vomiting, bleeding, severe bone marrow suppression
Hydrea (Hydroxyurea)	Melanoma, chronic myelocytic leukemia, head and neck cancer, advanced ovarian cancer	Bone marrow suppression, nausea, vomiting (less frequently), alopecia (rarely)
Purinethol (Mercaptopurine)	Acute lymphatic leukemia	Bone marrow suppression, liver toxicity, nausea and vomiting (uncommon)
Thioguanine	Acute nonlymphocytic leukemias	Bone marrow suppression, nausea, vomiting (infrequently)
ALKYLATING AGENTS		
BiCNU (carmustine)	Brain tumors, multiple myelomas, Hodgkin's disease, non-Hodgkin's lymphomas	Bone marrow suppression, bleeding, overwhelming infections, leukemia (after long use); infrequent pulmonary toxicity, nausea, vomiting
CeeNU (lomustine)	Brain tumors, Hodgkin's disease	Similar to BiCNU
Cytoxan (cyclophosphamide)	Malignant lymphomas, multiple myeloma, breast, ovarian cancer, neuroblastoma	Secondary malignancies, bone marrow suppression, alopecia, nausea, vomiting, cystitis, infertility, sterility, fetal harm
IFEX (ifosfamide)	Used adjunctively to treat testicular cancer	Hemorrhagic cystitis, nervous system toxicity, coma, bone marrow suppression, alopecia, nausea and vomiting
Alkeran (Melphalan)	Palliative treatment of multiple myeloma, ovarian cancer	Bone marrow suppression, secondary cancers
Mustargen (Mechlorethamine) (nitrogen mustard)	Hodgkin's disease, leukemias, lung cancer	Nausea and vomiting, bone marrow suppression, allergic reactions, immuno-suppression

Drug	Indicated use	Major side effects
Thiotepa	Breast, ovary, urinary bladder cancers	Bone marrow suppression (potentially fatal), nausea, vomiting, anorexia, sperm abnormalities
Myleran (busulfan)	Palliative treatment of chronic myelogenous leukemia	Bone marrow failure, pulmonary fibrosis (rare), secondary cancers, hyperpigmentation
Leukeran (chlorambucil)	Palliative treatment of chronic lymphatic leukemia, malignant lymphomas, Hodgkin's disease	Convulsions, infertility, leukemia, cancer, bone marrow suppression
PLANT ALKALOIDS		
Oncovin (vincristine sulfate)	Acute leukemia	Constipation, alopecia, muscle/nervous system weakness and disorders, anorexia, nausea, vomiting
Velban (vinblastine sulfate)	Hodgkin's disease, testicular cancer, Kaposi's sarcoma, lymphoma	Bone marrow suppression, alopecia, constipation, anorexia, nausea, vomiting, diarrhea, psychiatric disturbances, hypertension
PLATINUM COMPOUNDS		
Platinol (cisplatin)	Palliative treatment of testicular, ovarian and bladder cancers	Bone marrow suppression, renal toxicity, severe nausea and vomiting (frequent), potentially severe allergic reactions
Paraplatin (carboplatin)	Ovarian cancer	Bone marrow suppression, nausea, vomiting, possible secondary cancers.
HORMONES		
Emcyt (estramustine phosphate sodium)	Prostate cancer	Edema (swelling), heart attack (small incidence), nausea, vomiting, enlarged breasts and other estrogen-related side effects

Drug	Use	Side Effects
Estinyl (ethyl estradiol)	Prostate cancer; breast cancer in postmenopausal women	Estrogen-related effects including increased risk of cancer. Nausea and vomiting, headache, increase, decrease in weight
Estrace	Similar to Estinyl	
Lupron (leuprolide acetate)	Palliative treatment of prostate cancer	Edema, nausea, vomiting, (not frequent), hot flashes
Megace (megestrol acetate)	Breast, endometrium cancer	Weight gain, nausea, vomiting, bleeding, high blood sugar, alopecia
Sandostatin (octreotide acetate)	VIPomas	Nausea, diarrhea, abdominal pain, alopecia
Stilphostrol (diethylstilbestrol diphosphate)	Prostate cancer	Secondary cancers (after long-term use), thrombosis, potentially fatal benign liver tumors, hypertension, nausea, vomiting, anorexia, edema, nervousness. Other symptoms associated with oral contraceptives
TACE (chlorotrianisene)	Similar to Stilphostrol	
OTHER DRUGS		
Elspar (Asparaginase)	Acute lymphocytic leukemia	Frequent, unpredictable allergic reactions (possibly severe and fatal), pancreatitis, (possibly fatal), possibly fatal fever. Depression, hallucinations
VePesid (etoposide)	Small-cell lung cancer, testicular cancer	Bone marrow suppression, moderate nausea, vomiting, alopecia
Interferon	Hairy-cell leukemia, Kaposi's sarcoma	Flu-like symptoms, fatigue, anorexia, nausea, emotional problems

Source: Physicians' Desk Reference.

BECAUSE OF THE POSSIBILITY OF SERIOUS TOXIC RE-
ACTIONS, THE PATIENT SHOULD BE INFORMED BY
THE PHYSICIAN OF THE RISKS INVOLVED....DEATHS
HAVE BEEN REPORTED WITH THE USE OF
METHOTREXATE.[63]

Adriamycin, an equally toxic and potentially lethal cancer agent, is
commonly used to treat cancers of the bone, breast, ovaries, bladder,
thyroid, lung, and blood. The drug interferes with DNA synthesis and
also causes damage to chromosomes with a resultant mutation of
genes.[64]

Common side effects of Adriamycin include complete baldness,
acute and severe nausea and vomiting, inflammation of the stomach
and esophagus, ulceration and tissue death of the colon, potentially
fatal bleeding, and bone-marrow suppression. While these problems
are frightening, one of the drug's greatest dangers is the lethal effect it
may have on heart muscle. Fatalities can occur weeks after therapy has
been finished, and in some cases, life-threatening heart-rhythm
irregularities strike within hours after therapy.[65]

Recent data has also shown Adriamycin to deplete the body's stores
of vitamin C, leading to a drug-induced state of scurvy (see Chapter
6).

In an effort to improve the odds of a cure, doctors sometimes use
several drugs in combination with one another. "High-dose" chemotherapy regimens are also used to tip the scales in favor of a remission.
For example, in a treatment known as *leucovorin rescue*, patients are
flooded with potentially lethal doses of a folic-acid inhibiting drug and
then "rescued" by a neutralizing drug before fatal complications set
in.[66]

In the wake of such harsh and rigorous therapy, efforts are made to
minimize dangerous side effects. In fact, a primary skill of the
oncologist (or chemotherapist) lies in his or her ability to kill enough
of the cancer before killing the patient. To achieve this often delicate
balancing act, patients are carefully monitored in a hospital setting,
blood and urine tests are conducted frequently, and key indicators of
health are scrutinized to predict potentially catastrophic situations that
may arise. But even when patients are meticulously screened, deaths
still occur. For example, the antimetabolite drug 5-FU has such a
"narrow margin of safety" that it carries the following precaution:

Figure 4
Most Commonly Used Drugs to Treat Cancer (by Type)

Cancer Type	Drugs used to treat
Bone	Adriamycin, Methotrexate
Bladder	Adriamycin, Thiotepa, Platinol
Brain, Central nervous system (CNS)	BiCNU
Breast	Adriamycin, 5-FU, Cytoxan, Thiotepa, Estinyl, Megace, Teslac
Cervix	Blenoxane
Colon, rectum	5-FU
Head and neck	Blenoxane, Methotrexate, Hydrea
Hodgkin's disease	Adriamycin, BiCNU, Mustargen, Leukeran, Velban, Blenoxane
Kaposi's sarcoma	Velban, Interferon
Leukemias	Adriamycin, Daunorubicin, Methotrexate, Novantrone, Hydrea, Purinethol, Thioguanine, Myleran, Leukeran, Oncovin, Elspar, Interferon
Lymphomas	Adriamycin, BiCNU, Cytoxan, Leukeran, Velban, Blenoxane
Lung cancer	Adriamycin, Methotrexate, Mustargen, VePesid
Liver	FUDR (similar to 5-FU)
Melanoma	Hydrea
Multiple Myeloma	BiCNU, Cytoxan, Alkeran
Ovary	Adriamycin, Hydrea, Cytoxan, Thiotepa, Platinol
Pancreas	5-FU
Prostate	Emcyt, Estinyl, Lupron, Stilphostrol
Stomach, gastric	Mutamycin, 5-FU, Adriamycin
Testicle	Blenoxane, Plicamycin, IFEX, Velban, Platinol, VePesid
Thyroid	Adriamycin

> Fluorouracil (5-FU) is a highly toxic drug... severe hematological toxicity, gastrointestinal hemorrhage and even death may result from the use of Fluorouracil despite meticulous selection of patients and careful adjustment of dosage. Although severe toxicity is more likely to occur in poor-risk patients, fatalities may be encountered occasionally even in patients in relatively good condition.[67]

Physicians have come to accept such potentially lethal effects as the occupational hazards of chemotherapy. Highlighting this sentiment were doctors at Sloan-Kettering Cancer Center commonly heard referring to 5-FU and the cancer drug BiCNU, as "Five Feet Under" and "Be Seein' You" respectively.[68]

That dangerous adverse effects resulting from therapy occasionally occur and are not always predictable presents formidable anxieties and concerns for patients already suffering with the uncertainty of their illness. Adding to this quandary are the possibilities of such long-term complications as the growth of new cancers.

Like radiation, cancer drugs interfere with normal cellular function. The resultant aberrations may then trigger malignancy. But for some drugs, the chances of developing cancer may be greater than even the risks posed by radiation.

Studies have already shown that certain types of drugs can result in about a 2 percent cancer probability—even when the administered doses are low. Much higher doses are often used in actual treatment, however, and thus the *true* risks may be greater than suspected[69] Indeed, "many reports of acute leukemia" have been observed in patients being treated with specific anticancer agents.[70]

Proponents of drug therapy claim that a few days or weeks of distressing—even potentially dangerous—treatment is worth a life-time of cure. Unfortunately, not all drug courses are limited to days or weeks. For example, some cancer regimens may last up to a year, and the exhausting side effects they incur may seriously jeopardize patient compliance.[71]

The most common and agonizing side effects from drug therapy involve prolonged and severe nausea and vomiting; unless these are controlled, they may cause a serious deterioration in the quality of life. In an effort to control these symptoms and make treatments more bearable, clinicians prescribe antivomiting medicines known as *anti-*

emetics. However, for some highly toxic cancer drugs such as cisplatin, severe nausea still remains resistant to therapy.

Cisplatin, which is used to treat tumors of the testicles, ovaries, and bladder,[72] is so toxic that doctors are warned to avoid *external* contact with the drug by wearing gloves.[73] Severe gastrointestinal problems are almost a guaranteed reaction and despite the most potent anti-nausea medications in use, only half of the cisplatin patients taking them are helped.[74] A new class of antiemetics that block special "receptors" in the stomach have been shown to help a number of patients, but many remain symptomatic.[75]

The use of such highly dangerous and painful treatments might indeed be more tolerable if they were proven to cure cancer. Many drugs now in use however are not considered curative, but only a means of slowing down the inevitable growth of usually fatal tumors.

Are the use of such potentially dangerous treatments justified? Several outspoken critics do not think so and have even gone so far as to suggest that cancer treatment may actually *decrease* one's chance of survival.

As early as 1946, Dr. Stanley Reimann, director of research at Lankenau Cancer Hospital in Philadelphia, conducted a study which showed that cancer patients who did not receive surgery, radium, or X-ray therapy lived *longer* than those who had.[76] Several years later, Dr. Hardin Jones, a nationally prominent professor of medical physics and physiology at the University of California at Los Angeles delivered an equally shocking report to the 11th annual Science Writers Conference in New Orleans.[77]

Citing from an extensive analysis of a large population of cancer patients—some who were treated conventionally and others who had not received any treatment whatsoever—Dr. Jones stated that:

> Neither the timing nor the extent of treatment of [cancer] has appreciably altered the average course of the disease. The possibility exists that treatment makes the average situation worse.

Jones's claim was refuted by a federally sponsored study "proving" that patients who receive therapy fare better than those who do not. But Jones explained that statistical "trickery" was used in this study as a means of *guaranteeing* favorable results, whatever the true outcome.[78]

For example, Jones found that when cancer patients receiving treatment died before finishing a course of therapy, they were *excluded* from the final numbers appearing in the federal study. When patients in the untreated control group died, however, these deaths were *included* in the final numbers.[79]

After eliminating these biasing factors, Jones reported that the untreated cancer patients experienced the same life span as those receiving treatment. He told his New Orleans audience that it was "surprising" how similar the death rates really were for the two groups, adding that "the apparent life expectancy of untreated cases of cancer after [statistical] adjustment... seems to be greater than that of the treated cases."[80] In sum, Jones concluded his presentation by arguing that "the evidence for the falsity of claims about cancer therapy is overriding."

Although highly controversial and somewhat dated, Jones's conclusions have never been adequately discredited and have passed the scrutiny of three later studies.[81] In addition, other scientists have reached similar conclusions.

Dr. E. Cuyler Hammond, an epidemiologist** at the ACS, found that "a remarkable number of patients diagnosed with breast cancer in whom no evidence of breast cancer could be found later... received absolutely no treatment."[82] In another report, British investigators who studied the poor rate of cure for lung cancer noted that "no immediate treatment proved a significantly better policy for patient's survival and for the quality of remaining life."[83] And in a recent article appearing in *Scientific American*, a professor of microbiology at Harvard University noted that "the number of patients being cured can hardly amount to more than a few percent of those who are treated."[84]

In an effort to dissuade sagging public confidence, officials have launched a new campaign of optimism, promising that state of the art advances in research guarantee an imminent end to the epidemic of cancer plaguing the world. But three decades after Nixon's "war" on cancer was declared, the disease continues to claim a half-million American lives yearly. And by all accounts, that number appears to be increasing.

**Epidemiologists investigate the causes and control of diseases and epidemics among populations of people.

ONE

The Origins of the Alternative Therapy Movement

Interest in alternative medicine is not a new phenomenon. As early as 1825, homeopathy, a form of medicine essentially opposite to the drug-oriented method of treatment known as allopathy, began to take root. Other nontraditional methods also came into being, often in response to orthodox treatments seen as barbaric and unproductive. General anesthesia was not implemented until the mid-19th century, and up until that time surgery was commonly performed on cancer patients in varying degrees of consciousness. Even after the advent of anesthesia, surgical procedures were riddled with complications that often greatly diminished a patient's chances of survival, in spite of his illness.

A number of compassionate and dedicated healers, disgusted with the barbarism of surgery, devised their own noninvasive strategies for treating cancer; herbal formulas, immune-system stimulation, and the nutritional management of cancer were only a few of the many unconventional methods which marked the beginning of the alternative cancer therapy movement.

Whatever the ultimate worth of these early treatments, the established dictates of the day plagued their development. A careful review of the historic and scientific data reveals that such opposition was often a rule of principle rather than a matter of irrefutable, scientific investigation.

Numerous quack "cures" and remedies did surface throughout the 19th century and they were rightfully debunked. Other therapies that may have been legitimate, however, were not fully investigated and are still judged worthless. Many of these innovations were never subjected to conventional scrutiny because of protocol and procedural disagreements between biased reviewers and iconoclastic physicians. This disparity was usually enough to turn the tide of sentiment against the innovator.

In a number of cases, scientific research would later substantiate the condemned treatment long after the death of its proponent.

One of the earliest and most fascinating alternative cancer therapies originated on an Illinois farm in 1840. John Hoxsey, the farm owner, was struck by the behavior of a horse who had developed cancer on its hoof. According to anecdotal accounts, the animal's cancer was said to have disappeared after it ate herbs from a particular location on the pasture. An astute Hoxsey gathered up these herbs and concocted a formula from them. After claiming to cure sick animals with his remedy, Hoxsey began treating cancer in people and reported similar successes. The herbal remedy was then passed down through two generations of sons, the last of them Harry Hoxsey, who died in 1974.

Harry Hoxsey was a garish, colorful layman whose treatment attracted the interest of thousands of patients since the 1930s. Eventually, Hoxsey's self-proclaimed reputation as a curer of cancer, coupled with his lack of medical credentials, provoked the wrath of the medical establishment. Hoxsey was hounded by medical authorities for years, and then after investigators failed to corroborate his claims, he was forced to relinquish his practice.

Interestingly, while Hoxsey is generally regarded as one of this century's most blatant quacks, recent scientific studies have verified the antitumor, immune-enhancing properties of his formula's herbs (see chapter 10).

The use of herbs and other botanicals for cancer was not an exclusive invention of the Hoxsey family. In 1857, Dr. J. Weldon Fell announced the "successful" treatment of cancer with a Hoxsey-like preparation before key members of Middlesex Hospital in London. Fell's remedy was said to effect better results than surgery for some forms of cancer.[1] Doctors from Middlesex were impressed but did not agree with Fell that surgery could be replaced by his treatment. The Fell remedy eventually fell into disuse.

In 1858, Dr. John Pattison, a New York physician, also used a similar method to treat cancer. In addition, he gave his patients a salt-reduced diet consisting of fruits and vegetables.

Pattison was one of the first physicians to treat cancer as a constitutional disease, and he stressed the importance of whole-body care. He denounced surgery as a fate more terrible than the disease and emphasized strengthening the natural healing forces of the patient. But these concepts did not bode well with the medical establishment; despite Pattison's persistent requests, his method was never investigated.

Outrage at inhumane cancer treatment preoccupied the minds of many 19th-century clinicians. In Maurice Natenberg's classic text *The Cancer Blackout*, the brilliant London physician, Dr. Forbes Ross, wrote:

> A surgeon may spend his life carving his neighbor with astonishing facility and . . . may even write . . . of his superlative success as a cutter out of cancers . . . yet at the end of that man's life, although he has enjoyed a reputation as a good performer, he will have left nothing behind which will bring humanity . . . one iota near the true solution of the problem, the cause, therefore the cure of cancer.[2]

Like Fell and Pattison, Ross agreed that the entire constitution of the patient should be addressed before a cure could be achieved. Ross also stressed a more natural, vegetarian diet, and he may have been the first to observe a causal relationship between high-fat/low-fiber foods and cancer. But Ross did not negate the potential value of orthodox therapies and believed that surgery had merit.

At the turn of the century, traditional cancer therapy began to take shape. Surgery was followed by X-ray therapy and later, chemotherapy. However, a number of intrepid researchers continued exploring non-toxic treatment strategies designed to uphold the ancient medical edict "first do no harm." Remarkably, a few of these early treatment attempts yielded results whose ramifications would not be realized for many decades.

In 1891, the brilliant New York surgeon Dr. William Bradford Coley made what many now consider the first major breakthrough in cancer immunotherapy.

Coley became intrigued when a cancer patient completely recovered after being stricken with *erysipelas*—an acute skin infection. Believing there was a connection, Coley researched the literature and concluded that erysipelas had stimulated his patient's natural defenses to literally destroy malignant cells. After deliberately infecting patients with a germ-based vaccine, Coley managed to cure several cases of bone cancer nonsurgically—an astounding achievement at that time.

Throughout his career, Coley worked on developing the most effective toxins that would unleash an immunogenic response in his patients. He produced a number of vaccines that effected several astonishing remissions and cures.[3] Despite these reports, "Coley's toxins" (as they were later called) were not embraced by the scientific mainstream. Some historians now believe that Coley's work was overshadowed by vested interests in radium and pharmaceuticals to treat cancer.

After his death in 1936, Coley's daughter Helen Coley Naughts established a foundation dedicated to preserving her father's work. After compiling hundreds of scientific papers and over 850 case histories, the Nauts foundation reported that cure rates higher than 50 percent were being achieved with Coley's toxins for some forms of inoperable cancer.[4]

Later studies corroborated Coley's method and in 1976, it was removed from the list of worthless cancer remedies known as the *Unproven Therapies List* of the American Cancer Society (ACS). Today, Coley's toxins—now called *mixed bacterial vaccines*—are being used by a small number of immunotherapists, usually in conjunction with other naturally based modalities.

Dr. William Frederick Koch, another physician who proposed a nontoxic, immune-oriented strategy, was also rejected by his contemporaries.

Koch was a distinguished physician from Detroit who held various high-level posts throughout his tumultuous career. In 1917, he claimed that cancer resulted from a reduced amount of oxygen in the body's tissues caused by a buildup of poisons. He then developed *Glyoxilide*, a drug that could allegedly reverse the oxygen debt and inhibit cancer growth. Koch's theories were not unlike those formulated by Dr.

Joseph Gold, who in the 1960s, developed hydrazine sulfate, a controversial cancer drug that has recently been vindicated (see chapter 4).

The Detroit Medical Society agreed to evaluate Glyoxilide in a study involving seven cancer patients. But according to the official version, Koch was uncooperative and did not follow through with the proposed test. This led to a charge of insubordination and an unresolved trial.[5] Koch argued, however, that it was the medical society who had deliberately delayed testing, causing patients to worsen and forcing him to institute treatment independently.

In November of 1923, a hearing was convened by the Wayne County Medical Society to address the brewing allegations against Koch. At the hearing, physicians and patients testified on Koch's behalf and blamed the denouncement of Glyoxilide on loyalties to surgery and radium. One supporter, a Professor W. A. Dewey of the Department of Medicine, University of Michigan, complained that he had never observed such a biased charade in his "forty-four years" of medicine. In a letter to Koch, Dewey wrote:

> the composition of the [Medical Society] being for the most part surgeons and radium... 'experts', a class that assumes cancer to be curable only by these methods, was unfortunate.... no member of the committee was, in my opinion, qualified to sit in judgment on your treatment.[6]

The controversy over Glyoxilide was never effectively resolved, but later research did substantiate some of Koch's theories. In the 1930s, Nobel-prize winning physiologist Otto Warburg found that some cancer cells do, in fact, thrive in an oxygen-poor environment, as Koch had insisted. Years later, Dr. Albert Szent-Györgi, the discoverer of vitamin C, also credited Koch by calling him a pioneer in the field of free-radical cancer research.

While Coley and Koch paved the way for a more holistic view of cancer-treatment, another group of alternative doctors was blazing a different trail. In the tradition of Louis Pasteur, who was the first scientist to establish a germ theory for disease, these researchers believed that cancer was also an infectious disease caused by a germ or bacterium. They further proposed that cancer could be treated by helping the immune system launch an attack on the tumor-causing germs. This could be accomplished naturally and noninvasively by using a nontoxic vaccine.

If the "germ doctors" were correct, then the end of surgery and radium to treat cancer was near. But this presumption would not be taken lightly by the bastions of organized medicine. In fact, the cancer-germ controversy was to become one of the most protracted, bitter, and unresolved debates of modern medicine. And in light of current research and new data which has vindicated aspects of the theory, the controversy continues to linger.

In the early 1920s, a Canadian physician named Thomas Glover pioneered one of the first antibacterial vaccines designed to treat human cancer. In preliminary studies, several patients described as "hopeless" were reporting dramatic improvements in weight, appetite, and pain reduction.[7] In one case, a thirty-nine-year-old patient suffering from terminal breast cancer completely recovered after receiving vaccine treatment.[8] By 1925, Glover's germ theory gained further credibility after an independent study scientifically "proved" the connection between germs and cancer.[9]

Glover later organized a large vaccine trial involving several hundred advanced cancer patients at hospitals in Philadelphia.[10] According to a report later published in a leading medical journal, "favorable results [had] been secured [in the majority of these cases], and in some instances, the subjects [had] been discharged as symptom free...."[11] Amazingly, most of the trial patients were considered "incipient and hopeless" before treatment.[12]

Orthodox physicians remained skeptical of Glover's treatment results. According to historical accounts, news of the vaccine "cures" was said to have aroused "violent opposition" by medical experts antagonistic to an infectious theory of cancer. One of these experts was Dr. James Ewing, a nationally influential cancer scientist who argued that there was "no [germ] cause of cancer." Ewing cautioned that as soon as the public learned this fact, the less likely would they be "deceived by claims" such as those Dr. Glover made.[13] Meanwhile, Ewing proclaimed radium and surgery as the only truly effective means for treating cancer.

Despite this opposition, Glover steamed ahead with his research and treatment of patients, and by the late 1920s, a number of acutely ill people claimed to have been cured. Equally significant, laboratory evidence also emerged in support of the controversial vaccine.[14] But after a lengthy and politically charged dispute between Glover and officials of the Public Health Service, mainstream acceptance of the physician's unorthodox treatment stalled and his ideas eventually fell into disrepute.

Although the Glover controversy became an obscure footnote in the history of alternative cancer research, independent studies performed in America and Europe confirmed the cancer/germ link. While these studies were published in peer-approved scientific journals, they were still being ignored by the medical community.

In 1931, for example, Dr. Elise L'Esperance of Cornell University discovered a causative bacterium in Hodgkin's disease, a form of blood cancer. L'Esperance's discovery was then published in the highly regarded *Annals of Surgery*, but the report fell on deaf ears.[15] In 1941, the French physician George Mazet identified a leukemia-causing bacterium and he reported this discovery in the scientific journal *Montpellier Médecine*.[16] But again, orthodox researchers appeared unwilling to look into this potentially significant finding.

In wake of these and other reports,[17, 18, 19] a number of physicians began to treat patients with Glover-type vaccines, and many claimed favorable results. For example, the German physician Dr. Wilhelm von Brehmer announced numerous cancer remissions with an antibacterial vaccine. Dr. W. Mervyn Crofton of Ireland used an antitoxin derived from urine, and he also reported positive results. And in Italy, Clara Fonti treated a patient with stomach malignancy by first injecting *herself* with living cancer bacteria; when lesions developed, the physician transfused her own antibodies into the patient, who was then said to have dramatically improved. Dr. Fonti later developed a vaccine treatment and claimed hundreds of remissions.

In 1953, the long-term results of a vaccine trial involving 100 cancer patients were presented to the 6th International Congress of Microbiology in Rome by Dr. John E. White—a former Glover associate.[20] In White's landmark study, patients were followed for a twenty-seven-year period after finishing a course of vaccine therapy.

White reported that 67 percent of the vaccine patients showed no sign of cancer beyond the five-year waiting period after which a cure is generally denoted.* Particularly noteworthy, 58 percent of the patients described as either "hopeless" or "fair" before vaccine treatment

---

*This percentage is considerably higher than the current treatment rates for similar stages of cancer.

survived more than five years and in many cases, several decades after diagnosis was made. This percentage, if accurate, is also significantly higher than the response rates achieved via present-date treatments.

Despite corroboration of White's claims by a number of independent investigators, interest in the cancer-germ waned and as far as American scientists were concerned, the case on Glover was a closed issue. Orthodox cancer researchers were focusing, instead, on the "tried and true" methods to stem a growing incidence of cancer mortality. Postwar advances in surgery, coupled with new developments in radiation and drug therapies, promised new hope to a worried populace. Unfortunately, this effort did not bear fruit, as the dangerous upward spiral of cancer continued unchecked throughout the 1950s.

Most Americans still had faith that their medical institutions, buttressed by a new era of space-age technologies, would solve this growing cancer problem. But a few skeptical observers like Dr. Max Gerson were not convinced and stubbornly continued the search for more natural, humane alternatives.

Dr. Gerson had, like his 19th-century predecessors Ross and Pattison, devised a dietary treatment for cancer. But Gerson had taken the diet-therapy concept to heights never explored. His method consisted of organic, salt-free foods (that were supposed to reverse "toxic" imbalances in the body), massive amounts of raw pressed juices high in vitamin A, and special injections to help restore the "detoxifying" capabilities of the liver. Gerson brought medical evidence of his alleged cures before the U.S. Congress, but after a storm of controversy, the physician's license was revoked. Nonetheless, such notables as Albert Schweitzer esteemed Gerson, calling him one of "the eminent medical geniuses of the Twentieth century."

Years after Schweitzer's declaration, research would support Gerson's treatment concepts.

The German physician Joseph Issels also used a diet to combat cancer. But he pioneered what is considered the first eclectic treatment approach by using fever therapy, antibacterial vaccines, enzymes, oxygen/ozone treatments, and psychological counseling at a time when such methods were not even known to most orthodox practitioners—let alone subjects of scientific scrutiny.

In 1959, a Dutch statistician confirmed that Issels was achieving a remarkable 17 percent, five-year remission rate among patients with incurable cancers.[21] Despite this finding, Issels was arrested for his alleged role in urging patients to forego surgical treatment. The physician was prosecuted and sentenced to prison, but public outrage and the support of numerous patients forced a retrial. A second trial then ended in acquittal.

Although Issels had attracted a following, his methods continued to draw criticism. Eventually, sentiment turned against Issels after an Olympic athlete suffering from incurable colon cancer sought the physician's help and later died.[22]

While the European medical orthodoxy was sitting in judgment on Issels, American cancer experts were again doing battle—this time with the maverick physician Dr. Andrew Ivy. Ivy's nontoxic cancer drug *Krebiozen* was considered one of the most notorious examples of quackery this century, and it provoked a bitter and highly publicized debate that was never satisfactorily resolved.

The ACS admitted that Ivy was "a legitimate ... research scientist" but added that he "sacrificed his career and reputation to promote a make-believe cancer cure."[23] The facts, however, paint a completely different picture of the controversial scientist.

According to the American Physiological Society, Ivy had authored a remarkable 1,441 medical papers and was considered the most cited research scientist in the world.[24] He served as a director for both the Naval Medical Research Institute and the National Advisory Cancer Council, represented the Allies as a medical authority during the Nuremberg trials and later as president of the ACS itself.

Ivy's sparkling credentials were unparalleled and most likely surpassed the stature of most alternative as well as orthodox physicians. And yet, his endorsement of an innovative and conceptually unique treatment embroiled him in a vicious, lengthy battle that ended in his rejection by the medical community.

Ivy's problems began when he tested Krebiozen on cancer patients and reported a number of dramatic cures and remissions with it. Krebiozen (which is made from horse blood immunogenically stimulated with a tuberculosislike organism) was said to have a regulatory effect on abnormal cells. An investigation by the American Medical Association and the Food and Drug Administration (FDA) failed to corroborate this claim despite an absence of clinical trials which Ivy had continually requested. As the controversy intensified, allegations of conspiracy to defraud Ivy's findings and counterallegations of impropriety and unethical practice against the physician were leveled.

Still, the ACS had expressed a willingness to screen Krebiozen, but protocol disagreements between Ivy and government scientists stalled proposed testing. Then in 1963, the FDA formally announced that Krebiozen was, in fact, nothing more than *creatine*, an ordinary, nontherapeutic substance found in muscle tissues. To support its claim, the FDA released a spectrograph showing that Krebiozen and creatine were essentially the same thing.**

When the spectrographs were carefully reexamined by a leading scientific authority, however, twenty-nine color differences between Krebiozen and creatine were actually found.[25] Evidently, the spectrographs were either mistakenly or deliberately misaligned so that Krebiozen and creatine appeared to share points of similarity; when the images were realigned, obvious differences were noted.[26]

Despite this revelation, the negative publicity surrounding Krebiozen was so intense that an appropriately conducted trial never did materialize. Ivy then formed his own *Ivy Research Institute* and, after unsuccessfully trying to generate interest in Krebiozen, died in 1978.

Interestingly, while Krebiozen is generally considered a "phony" cancer drug, it is made from the same class of bacteria used in the conventional cancer drug actinomycin-D. The major difference is that Krebiozen is a nontoxic substance derived from the immune system of horses; actinomycin-D, on the other hand, is an antibiotically derived drug that is highly toxic and sometimes lethal.

In wake of the ill-fated Krebiozen affair, scientific tolerance toward alternative cancer treatments became increasingly short-fused. Fueling this intolerance was a growing interest in the use of toxic chemicals to treat cancer. Because the profit potential predicted for cancer drugs was enormous, private industry began pouring millions of dollars into research during the Fifties and Sixties. This decision was a lucrative one. By the 1990s, millions of cancer patients throughout the world were being treated by an armament of drugs at a cost of billions of dollars yearly.

The push to test and develop cancer drugs was actually a legacy championed by the petrochemical industry in the early 1920s. Because crude oil and its derivatives were essential to the synthesis of drugs, one of the petrochemical industry's leading priorities was to control and influence world production of pharmaceuticals. Inevitably, this influence helped to shape a *philosophy* of cancer therapy that gradu-

---

**Spectrograms are used to measure the spectral wavelengths unique to different substances; similar substances share similar spectrographic characteristics.

ally became drug-oriented. Shortly after World War I, the marriage of medicine and industry occurred on a grand scale when I. G. Farben, the German cartel giant with large holdings in oil, began to purchase large assets of the American drug industry. In 1962, Farben's assets were sold and such dynasties as the Rockefellers took over many of the holdings, including pharmaceuticals. This overlapping of interests insured that scientific as well as economic forces were shaping the direction of American cancer research.

It is now commonplace to find members of industry sitting on the boards of universities and cancer centers. These key players influence the design of medical school curricula and are instrumental in the decision-making process involving research. Indeed, this conflict of interest has had a predictable and stifling effect on such areas as grant approval for novel and innovative avenues of study. It has also created a preordained, unyielding bias against nondrug, holistically oriented cancer therapies.

TWO

Gerson's Diet Therapy

The Gerson therapy, named after Max Gerson, M.D., is based on the premise that cancer results from a degeneration of the human body brought on by improper eating and cooking practices common to modern civilization. Specifically, treatment is aimed at correcting these "deficiencies" by preparing and consuming foods in as close to their natural state as possible.

In the Gerson diet, salt is prohibited and potassium-rich foods are emphasized. Patients are also given iodine, liver, and other compounds believed to help the immune system. Enemas are also administered as a means of "detoxifying" or ridding the body of toxins believed to play a role in the cancer process.

In the 1950s, the Gerson therapy was placed on the *Unproven Therapies List* of the American Cancer Society (ACS). Dr. Gerson died in 1959 and shortly afterward, his daughters established a clinic in Tijuana, Mexico, to carry on their father's work.

At this time, the Gerson Clinic continues operating in Mexico. In addition to offering a diet program, the clinic also treats patients with other "holistic" therapies, including the controversial cancer drug Laetrile, vaccines, vitamins, and "ozone" therapy which is purported to destroy infections and promote normal healing.

Gerson Clinic physicians suggest that patients stay between three to eight weeks in their Mexican facility. The cost of treatment is estimated at $495 per day.

Max Gerson's Credentials

Dr. Max Gerson was born in 1881, in the German town of Wongrowitz. He received his medical education at the universities of Breslau, Würzburg, Berlin, and Freiburg and later trained with world-renowned physiologists and physicians before establishing a medical practice in Bielefeld, Germany.[1]

In 1942, Gerson became a U.S. citizen and after passing his medical boards, practiced in New York City's Gotham Hospital.[2] There, he treated cancer patients with his unusual diet regimen.

How Dr. Gerson Developed His Cancer Therapy

As a young internal medicine and neurology specialist, Dr. Gerson often suffered from recurrent bouts of migraine headache so severe that he would become bedridden for days. Convinced that his headaches were the result of an improper diet, Gerson eliminated meat, salt, fats, and other foods he believed were "toxic." Through this unusual program, the young German doctor reportedly cured his problem and began treating other migraine patients accordingly. Oddly, one of these patients claimed that in addition to his headaches subsiding, his skin tuberculosis had also vanished. This was a potentially important finding because sulfa drugs to treat TB had not yet been developed.

Believing that he had stumbled onto something significant, Gerson began treating a large number of people with skin TB and reported dramatic results. In 1929, after clinical trials were conducted in Munich, Kassel, and Berlin, the famous German surgeon Sauerbach announced that Gerson's treatment cured 446 out of 450 people with skin TB.[3] These findings were then published in several peer review journals in Germany.[4, 5]

A demonstration of Gerson's TB successes was to be held by the Berlin Medical Association. But because of the growing political unrest in Germany, in March 1933 Gerson emigrated to Paris, where he continued his practice and dietary research. Several years later, he treated a number of desperately ill cancer patients with his diet and claimed that three out of seven responded favorably.[6] Gerson then spent the next several years intensively researching the relationship between cancer growth and diet.

Scientific Evidence to Support Dr. Gerson's Dietary Treatment

Early in his research, Dr. Gerson discovered reports which showed a direct relationship between tumor shrinkage and diet.[7, 8, 9] In one independent study, German scientists directly influenced the outcome of certain types of liver cancer in rats by simply lowering fat intake and limiting the diet to specific vegetables.[10] These investigators concluded[11] that:

> no tumor has been found that does not respond to a restricted diet... the inhibition [of foods] involved both a decrease in the total number of tumors and a delay in the average time of appearance.

Gerson incorporated these findings into his own diet program and was later influenced by the pioneering research of Nobel-prize winning biochemist Otto Warburg.

In the 1930s, Warburg claimed that cancer cells thrive in an environment having little or no oxygen.[12] According to Warburg, conditions in the human body which reduce the oxygenation of cells and tissues are fodder for the growth of cancer. In his classic treatise *The Prime Cause and Prevention of Cancer*, Warburg proposed that an improper utilization of minerals and vitamins and a toxic physical state might contribute to a lowering of oxygen in the body's cells with the ultimate result being cancer.[13]

Drawing upon Warburg's research, Gerson felt that organically grown foods rich in oxygen-promoting enzymes which could "cleanse" or "detoxify" the body were necessary to help rid the body of cancer. These foods include fruits, vegetables, and complex carbohydrates. Much emphasis was also placed on drinking twelve or more glasses of raw pressed juices daily. Milk, cheese, butter, fish, and eggs were excluded during the initial stages of therapy (see Figure 1).

Dr. Gerson also believed that dangerous food-processing techniques and other unhealthy dietary practices common to modern civilization had resulted in a dangerous increase of sodium in the diet. In Gerson's view, an excess of sodium causes a deficiency of potassium in the body and this imbalance may disrupt the normal function of cells, thereby precipitating cancer. He thus believed that by eliminating salt and increasing the intake of potassium, a favorable outcome in cancer treatment could be achieved.[14]

The Importance of the Liver in Gerson's Treatment

Gerson cited earlier research showing a link between cancer growth and a weakened liver.[15] He also felt that cancer was a disease caused by a constant state of "toxicity" or poisoning existing in the body. Since the liver rids the body of toxins and other unhealthy substances, Gerson felt that its optimum function was paramount to the healing of cancer.[16]

The Rationale Behind Coffee Enemas

Experiments conducted by German scientists in 1923 had shown that caffeine could open up the bile ducts and veins in the liver, resulting in better circulation to that organ and an improvement in its function.[17, 18] As a result, Gerson believed that coffee, introduced in the form of enemas, could stimulate this process. Some current research has further substantiated the rationale for using enemas in cancer treatment.[19]

Gerson also claimed that because his diet could literally dissolve tumors in a matter of weeks or even days, enemas were essential for the removal of poisons released into the body from large, dying masses of cancer cells. Without this removal, explained the physician, coma and death could occur.

Dr. Gerson Announces His Medical Concepts to Colleagues

While at Gotham, Gerson actively shared his theories and treatment ideas with colleagues, including Dr. George Miley, the director-in-chief of the hospital. Initially, Miley was skeptical and called Gerson's

Figure 1
The Gerson Diet for Cancer

PROHIBITED FOODS:

avocados	salt and all substitutes
berries	refined, salted, smoked foods
commercial beverages	sulfured foods
candy	fat
cake	white enriched flour
chocolate	nuts
cocoa	oil
coffee, tea	spices (pepper, paprika)
cream	pineapples
cucumbers	sugar (white refined)

soy beans and products
drinking water (to allow maximum absorption of fruit juices).

PROHIBITED ITEMS, OTHER:

nicotine
alcohol
bottled, canned, preserved
or frozen foods
fluorine
Epsom salts

TEMPORARILY FORBIDDEN FOODS

butter	fish
cheese	meat
eggs	milk

NECESSARY FOODS

fruit
juices of fruit, vegetables, and leaves
vegetables, salads
special soup
potatoes
oatmeal, bread etc.

GERSON SAMPLE DIET:

BREAKFAST

1 glass juice
large portion oatmeal
bread, dark rye, toasted or plain with honey or stewed fruit (no preserves).

LUNCH

Salad (raw food)
Pot cheese and buttermilk (as prescribed)
1 glass warm soup
1 glass juice
large baked potato
vegetables, cooked
dessert: fruit, stewed or raw

DINNER

salad (raw food)
pot cheese and buttermilk (as prescribed)
1 glass warm soup
1 glass juice
large baked potato
2 vegetables, cooked
dessert: raw or stewed fruit

HOURLY JUICE SCHEDULE

TIME	JUICE	DIET	COFFEE ENEMAS
08:00	Orange	Breakfast	Every four hours or more as needed
09:00	Green*		
10:00	Apple-carrot		
11:00	Liver		
12:00	Green		
1:00	Apple-carrot	Lunch	
2:00	Green		
3:00	Liver		
4:00	Liver		
5:00	Apple-carrot		
5:30	Apple-carrot		
6:00	Green		
7:00	Apple-carrot	Dinner	

Source: The Gerson Institute, Bonita, California

*Green leaf juice consists of a variety of ground vegetable leaves including lettuce, red cabbage, escarole, green pepper, and watercress.

method "fantastic" but later "completely logical."[20] Dr. Charles Bailey, one of this century's most renowned chest surgeons, was invited to visit Gerson in 1942, and after reviewing patient data, expressed surprise at the "cures" that had been reported.[21] And the physician who shared Gerson's offices in New York City reported that some patients with inoperable breast, stomach, lung, and brain cancers had indeed, made remarkable recoveries.[22]

Gerson's Most Publicized Patient

In the 1940s, Dr. Gerson began treating a sixteen-year-old boy named John Gunther. Gunther, who had been diagnosed with an inoperable brain tumor and given only a few weeks to live, actually survived another eight months on Gerson's program. This recovery was said to have astounded doctors.

The most detailed account of John Gunther's plight was chronicled in the classic work *Death Be Not Proud*, written by his father, a critically acclaimed journalist.[23]

Mr. Gunther explained that despite a series of X-ray treatments and surgery, his son's tumor continued to grow at a "monstrous pace." After being given a prognosis of only weeks to live, the Gunther family consulted Gerson, who then ordered his young patient to stop taking all drugs because they were considered toxic to the body and especially the liver. In addition to a strict diet, the boy received frequent coffee enemas along with liver and spleen injections.

After a few months, John Gunther was reported to have made an "astounding" recovery. In fact, pathologists confirmed that he was *free* from active cancer. According to the boy's father, "doctor after doctor" examined him and expressed "their free amazement."[24] Gunther was said to have then enjoyed a quality of life practically impossible before commencing diet therapy, and in the spring of his "cure" graduated from high school. Yet the ACS contended that Gunther's recovery was probably brought about by a "delayed reaction" to conventional treatments the boy had received earlier.

On June 22, 1947, eight months after doctors had labeled him "hopeless," Gunther died from a recurrence of his cancer. Despite the loss, John Gunther Sr. had become one of Gerson's most ardent supporters and he was convinced that "beyond a reasonable doubt... [Gerson's] diet did effect...cures."[25]

Gerson was deeply affected by the boy's death and later offered an explanation as to why the cancer had returned. At a lecture given in Escondido, California, in 1956, Gerson revealed that while still on diet therapy, Gunther was given a pituitary hormone by his family doctor for an eczema condition. Gerson initially resisted the idea fearing the tumor would regrow, but then yielded. Shortly thereafter, the boy's cancer did return and Gerson lamented that for a long time, he "couldn't sleep nights" because of the blunder. Afterward, the physician modified his treatment approach and banned the use of any hormones during cancer treatment. Recent research has shown a direct correlation between pituitary hormone use and brain cancer.[26, 27]

Government Funding for Gerson's Therapy

In July 1946, Gerson appeared before a select Congressional subcommittee headed by Claude Pepper (D) of Florida.[28] The bill being reviewed, which would appropriate money for various avenues of cancer research, was entitled S.1875.

Gerson presented five "cured" patients along with their medical records and pathology reports before and after therapy. Further, a number of Gerson's fellow physicians, including Dr. Miley, testified on his behalf.

The first patient testified under oath that he had "seen patients who appeared to be so far gone as to be beyond the pale of anything but miracles. These miracles are in fact being performed by Max Gerson M.D., 815 Park Avenue, New York."[29] The man also reported that Gerson completely cured a friend's inoperable lung cancer.

A woman from Hillside, New Jersey, who had been treated by Gerson explained that she had been diagnosed with a spinal cord tumor that could not be surgically removed. Since the tumor began to spread into various nerve networks, doctors warned family members that paralysis would soon strike and that the prognosis would eventually prove fatal. Doctors urged that the woman be made "as comfortable as possible" since they could do nothing else to save her.[30]

Six months after receiving Gerson's treatment, the woman apparently regained nearly full use of her limbs which were weakened by her condition. Her doctors confirmed that the cancer had been arrested. To corroborate this recovery, Pepper called the woman's physician to the stand. "Is it your opinion that the apparent cure . . . in the condition of [the patient] which you witnessed is due to [Gerson's treatment]?" asked Pepper. The doctor, who consulted with a neurologist from Columbia University before finalizing his conclusions, replied that he could not "see anything else to account for it . . . it [is not] a coincidence."[31]

Another patient, a woman from Pennsylvania, had been riddled with cancer; tumors infiltrated her bowels, branched toward vessels near her heart, and were beginning to colonize in her liver. Surgery, other than for the purpose of inserting a drainage bag, was ruled out. According to surgeons, it was "very definite that she would not live very long."[32]

Having heard of Gerson, the woman was brought to Gotham for treatment. One month later, X-rays showed no evidence of cancer.[33] The woman's personal physician claimed to "have never witnessed anything like it." Other specialists associated with the case were equally impressed and a pathologist who reviewed the patient's records called the woman "cured" with "no evidence of the original growth."[34]

Doctors who had an opportunity to review Gerson's therapy also testified.

Dr. Miley commended Gerson and insisted that his method offered a "new approach to the cancer problem." Miley reported that the diet effected a 90 percent reduction in pain, blocked the spread of some cancers, and appeared to control infections that normally result from the disease.[35] The physician urged Congress that:

> in view of the success so far and the excellent future promise of the Gerson [method] it would be unthinkable not to give major consideration to this new avenue of approach to the cancer problem in the research program contemplated by bill S.1875.

Four other physicians from Gotham submitted sworn statements to the Congressional panel:[36]

> J.V.R., M.D., New York, June 29, 1946: While all of (the cancer patients) did not respond...the favorable results in some were very striking...I believe this type of treatment should be investigated intensively.

> H.S.H., M.D., New York, June 27, 1946: I have observed several cases of malignancy which have been apparently arrested by the Gerson diet....

> C.P.B., M.D., New York, June 27, 1946: ...I have closely followed the cases of malignancy under treatment by the Gerson diet...I have been much impressed by the apparent reduction of

the tumor in several cases and the marked clinical improvement of the others. There certainly is a definite benefit in many instances...the research must be continued along these lines.

A.L.W., M.D., New York, June 28, 1946: It is my carefully considered opinion that many of these patients have greatly benefited...the method should be given an intensive trial.

The Outcome of Gerson's Congressional Hearing

According to Congressional records, the Gerson cancer therapy lost Senate approval for research appropriation by one vote. Various theories have emerged to explain why this conclusion was reached.

Some noted observers feel that vested interests in chemotherapy, a rapidly growing specialty toward the end of the 1940s, overshadowed interest in Gerson's nondrug treatment method.[37] Others have suggested that a conflict of interests stemming from Claude Pepper's ties to the ACS may have biased the voting.[38]

But an article appearing in the *Journal of the American Medical Association* (JAMA) in 1946 simply concluded that there was not enough evidence to warrant an investigation into the controversial treatment.[39] Shortly after the *JAMA* article, further "investigations" also concluded that Gerson's method was "without benefit."

For example in 1947, the NCI reviewed the records of ten patients treated by Gerson and found "no evidence" of improvement. The NCI's conclusions however, were apparently not due to a lack of benefit from Gerson's treatment; rather, the NCI admitted that it was "impossible" to properly evaluate the patients because all had received prior therapies and these could have biased any conclusions.[40] Despite this admission, the NCI still officially concluded that the Gerson treatment was without merit.

In addition, the ACS states that many of the patients treated and later "cured" by Gerson during the 1940s may have not had cancer in the first place. According to a special investigative committee, there existed "no case in which...a cure of malignant disease has been obtained by [Gerson's] treatment."[41] But defenders of Gerson have argued that his patients definitely had cancer and these were all confirmed by needle biopsy, X-ray reports, and the most effective diagnostic techniques available at that time.[42] These diagnoses were also reportedly made by physicians or hospitals independent of Gerson.[43]

By 1950, Gerson's therapy was considered ineffective against cancer and was therefore officially banned in the United States.

The Gerson Clinic Today

The ACS reported in 1990 that thirteen people receiving the Gerson therapy in Tijuana, Mexico, experienced treatment-related infections.[44] Ten of the infections were apparently caused by improperly sterilized equipment used in liver injections and three others by microorganisms transmitted through enemas.[45]

The ACS also cites two examples of people dying from complications related to the use of enemas. One of these cases involved a forty-six-year-old woman who took 10 to 12 coffee enemas one night as part of her treatment. Another patient apparently died after experiencing a "fluid and electrolyte" imbalance believed caused by enemas.*[46]

The first woman, who was not under proper medical supervision, did not adhere to Gerson's regimen, which prescribes no more than one enema every two hours for a maximum of twelve per day.[47] But while the ACS implicates enemas as the primary source of trouble in this woman's case, her actual cause of death was from pneumonia and *low potassium* levels. (The ACS does not explain *how* this woman developed low potassium levels in view of the fact that Gerson's therapy is known to *overload* the body with this mineral).

The second person died from an electrolyte imbalance. After leaving the clinic in "good health," the patient returned home, continued to treat herself without "seeing a local physician" and then later died from apparent complications. Defenders of the Gerson therapy point out that this scenario could easily have been avoided if proper medical supervision was in place.

Supporting Clinical Evidence for the Gerson Method

Although the ACS has officially concluded that "no supporting" evidence shows any efficacy from the Gerson treatment,[48] two scien-

*Electrolytes are chemicals needed by the cells for proper functioning. Electrolyte imbalances can be caused by dehydration or severe diarrhea.

tific papers corroborating diet as a means of treating cancer had already appeared in both Great Britain and Austria prior to the ACS's conclusion.

The first paper, published in the noted British medical journal *Lancet*, describes a study conducted by British cancer specialists who visited the Gerson clinic in 1989.[49] Because patient records were destroyed in a fire several years earlier, the investigators were able to review only a limited amount of data regarding treatment results.[50]

The British scientists were also informed that patients and their families often did not report back to the clinic on their progress.[51] Adding to this dilemma was the fact that many of these patients had already received standard cancer therapies before their visits to Mexico; this factor could have marred any objective interpretation of the diet treatment. As a result, the British researchers concluded that the Gerson therapy was not entirely "assessable."[52]

Despite these difficulties, the investigators did note a particularly "intriguing" feature of the diet: its effect on pain. Although many patients had "extensive" cancer throughout their bodies and were thoroughly dependent on morphine and other drugs, the diet regimen almost entirely eliminated the need for such medication. Moreover, the British admitted that in spite of protocol difficulties, "definite tumor regression" could be documented in some patients.[53]

The second study, conducted by a team of Austrian surgeons in 1984, is perhaps more significant because it involved the actual testing of diet therapy in a clinical setting.[54] The only drawback was that the researchers combined both diet therapy with drugs and other conventional treatments for cancer. This regimen naturally made a final evaluation of Gerson's method impossible and also sharply contradicted his position that drugs damage and interfere with the cleansing process of the liver. Further complicating matters, the Austrian doctors did not faithfully adhere to Gerson's diet but instead, revised it. In spite of these variables, several highly favorable results were still reported.

One seventy-seven-year-old woman with advanced cancer experienced a *complete* remission, which the researchers attributed solely to diet treatment. In another case, a man suffering from malignant cancer of the lymphatic system developed a serious liver condition, which threatened his chances for recovery. Diet therapy completely normalized his liver and allowed him to continue with the medical regimen he had been receiving. He then went into remission.

Overall, the Austrian researchers were able to arrive at some definite conclusions by studying two groups of patients: those who volunteered for the diet treatment versus those who chose no therapy at all. In all cases, the participants were considered terminal before starting the trial.

Since the patients in the controlled study had advanced cancer and were beyond the hope of curability, an accurate evaluation of diet therapy would seem inconclusive at best. But in spite of this consideration, the diet-treated group lived an average of *one year longer* than their nontreated counterparts. While the Austrian researchers were cautious and admitted that their patient group was small, they did emphasize that the positive responses could "only be seen as a trend."

After completing their six-year study, the Austrians officially reported that several favorable results could be "traced back to diet therapy." For example:

—*cachexia*, which is the devastating wasting-away syndrome associated with cancer, was, in most cases, reversed

—*pain medication* (as noted by the British doctors and colleagues of Gerson during the Congressional testimony) was reduced and even eliminated

—tumor growth in certain organs was slowed down and the avoidance of other complications—such as dangerous fluid buildup associated with tumors—directly attributed to the "therapeutic success of the dietary regimen."[55]

The researchers concluded that:

the preliminary results reported...encourage us to continue and...to intensify the use of dietary therapy measures, and we are seeking intensive cooperation with all those who are experienced in this at present still highly controversial area of work.[56]

In the most recent report on Gerson's method, *JAMA* cites a number of flaws that are supposed to invalidate the controversial therapy.[57] But as is often the case in alternative medicine, "evidence" can differ significantly depending on *which* report one ascribes to.

For example, one key point brought up in the *JAMA* article is that the roasted, ground coffee used by Gerson practitioners in their enema preparations does not contain two essential ingredients active in cleansing out the liver; only green coffee beans contain these two chemicals. According to this argument, coffee enemas do not possess any therapeutic activity at all. However, the Austrian researchers admitted that, while ground coffee has less of the key ingredients than green coffee beans, enemas made from ground coffee still show activity in the liver. In fact, the Austrians concluded that in lieu of further research, they were forced to continue using enemas as Gerson had recommended to achieve the desired therapeutic results.

While the rationale for coffee enemas (and other aspects of the Gerson treatment) are disputed for *scientific* reasons, the *objective* alleviation of intense, morphine-dependent pain (and other parameters of well-being) in thousands of patients is not addressed; in addition, *JAMA* does not quote from or review even briefly the human studies which do show favorable therapeutic results from diet therapy.

The only scientific trial to date remains the Austrian study. Though not an exact representative of Gerson's actual treatment, this study offers clinical evidence that diet can benefit cancer patients. While any absolute conclusions would be premature, it would likewise be presumptuous to suggest that no data exists whatsoever showing a connection between diet as a potential therapy for some forms of cancer.

Until a long-term, controlled study of Gerson's actual therapy is conducted, however, definite conclusions about its effectiveness will remain open to speculation.

For further information contact:

The Gerson Institute
P.O. Box 430
Bonita, CA 91908
(619) 472-7450

THREE

The Livingston Therapy

D_{r.} Virginia Livingston, a highly controversial physician, believed that cancer was an infectious disease caused by a tuberculosis-like germ.

As a result of her research, Livingston developed a treatment that she claimed could target infectious cancer germs. This treatment included vaccines made from patients' body fluids, vitamins, and minerals to help boost the immune system and a prohibitive diet designed to "detoxify" the body and help the liver function more efficiently.

Virginia Livingston died in 1990, and her clinic is now under the supervision of Dr. Kenneth C. Forror. Treatment still includes diet, vitamins and other immunity-enhancing strategies. Livingston's original vaccine, however, has been banned by the state of California.[1]

At this time, the American Cancer Society (ACS) disputes the Livingston therapy and has placed it on the *Unproven Therapies List*.

Virginia Livingston's Credentials

The late Dr. Virginia Livingston received her Bachelors Degree in Science from Vassar College and in 1936 graduated from the New York University School of Medicine—one of the school's few female graduates at that time.[2] She then became one of the first female medical residents ever assigned to a hospital in New York City's history.[3] In 1949, Livingston was elected chief of the Presbyterian Hospital Laboratory for the Study of Proliferative Diseases at Rutgers University.[4] Later, she established an allergy and immunology practice in San Diego and became a member in good standing of the San Diego Medical Association.

How Livingston Discovered the "Cancer Germ"

While working as a school physician in 1947, Livingston examined a nurse suffering from a rare skin condition. Samples of the nurse's skin tissues revealed clusters of germs which Livingston could not identify. Later, when these germs were injected into guinea pigs, the animals developed cancerous lesions. Because cancer normally afflicts only one in every half-million guinea pigs, Livingston deduced that the infectious germs might be causing the cancer.[5] As a consequence of this chance discovery, Livingston became intent on finding a possible relationship between germs and cancer.

After being assigned to the Presbyterian Hospital Laboratory, Livingston actively began studying cancerous tissues taken from surgical patients and repeatedly claimed to find evidence of bacterial organisms. To better determine what these germs were, Livingston used a process known as "staining." (Specific germs can be identified by the different colored stains they absorb). Because the microbes infesting her specimens were staining red, Livingston announced that they bore a close resemblance to the organisms of tuberculosis and leprosy which also take on a reddish stain.

How Livingston "Proved" Her Theory

Dr. Livingston and her long-time associate Dr. Eleanor Alexander-Jackson, a noted scientist and authority on tuberculosis, subjected the "cancer germ" to a set of scientific laws known as *Koch's postulates*. The time-honored postulates, which prove a cause and effect between a specific germ and disease, involve the following four steps:

1. The suspected germ must be consistently found in all animals suffering from a particular disease

2. The germ must be "cultured" (i.e., allowed to grow) on an artificial medium outside of the animal
3. Inoculation of the germ into healthy animals must produce the same disease
4. The germ must then be recovered from the newly infected animal.

In 1950, Livingston and Jackson announced that they had, in fact, fulfilled Koch's postulates, establishing a definite link between cancer and tuberculosis-like bacteria. They then published the result of this finding in the *American Journal of the Medical Sciences*.[6]

Three years later, Livingston and Jackson presented their findings to the Sixth International Congress of Microbiology in Rome.[7]

Livingston Names the Cancer Germ

At a scientific meeting in 1969, Livingston formally classified and named the infectious cancer-causing germ *Progenitor cryptocides* (prō-jene'ter krip' tō-sīd-ēz). This organism was considered a "close cousin" of the germs that cause leprosy and tuberculosis.[8]

How Livingston Developed a Cancer Vaccine

Livingston's first vaccine was made by inoculating human cancer bacteria into healthy animals; after the inoculations caused the animals' immune systems to make antibodies, these were extracted and purified into a serum. This serum was later given to chickens afflicted with cancer and apparently near death.[9] One day after treatment, the chickens began showing signs of recovery, and later several were reportedly cured.[10]

After reporting her finding, Livingston was contacted by a hospital volunteer in San Diego whose husband had been diagnosed with an inoperable tumor. Hearing of Livingston's vaccine successes with animals, the woman felt a similar treatment might offer her husband some hope.[11] Livingston agreed to treat the man.

Altering the method she used in her earlier animal experiments, Livingston made a vaccine from bacteria found in her patient's urine. This type of treatment is known as *autogenous vaccine therapy*, and it is based on the earlier pioneering work of Dr. W. Mervyn Crofton of Ireland.[12] (The rationale behind such a therapy is that disease-causing germs which are unique to an individual will be more effective at stimulating that individual's immune system). After a few weeks on the vaccine, the man's tumor reportedly shriveled away to nothing. He then died twenty years later of natural causes.[13]

Another of Livingston's first reported cures was that of a cancer physician named Owen Webster Wheeler, a prestigious member of the San Diego medical community for thirty years and also a cofounder of Doctors Hospital in that city.[14]

In 1972, Dr. Wheeler discovered a lump in his neck while shaving, and tests revealed that he had inoperable cancer. Colleagues advised radiation and chemotherapy as Wheeler's only hope because his tumor—described as the "size of a lemon"—had encroached on delicate nerves and blood vessels and would soon prove fatal. But Wheeler was convinced that standard treatment could not help him. Risking the criticism of colleagues and the possibility of not benefiting from conventional therapy, he chose Livingston's treatment solely. After six months on the vaccine and diet regimen, the physician reported that his otherwise fatal cancer had been completely cured.[15]

Livingston and Jackson then conducted a trial of their vaccine and diet therapy involving forty cancer patients. They later reported in a medical journal that "a number" of the patients "appeared to be improving" but cautiously pointed out that a larger trial would have to be conducted before their results could become conclusive.[16]

Livingston and Her Clinic

Livingston's clinic, located in San Diego, was established in 1970. Treatment originally included autogenous vaccines, which are now banned; antibiotics, vitamins, minerals, and a diet similar to the one used in the Gerson therapy are still being used.

The Livingston diet allows only unprocessed fruits, vegetables, herbs, nuts, and other organic foods. Salt, saturated fats, meats and most dairy products are prohibited (see Figure 1). Chicken is also banned because Livingston believed that minute, viruslike forms of the cancer germ commonly infect poultry and can be transmitted to humans. This claim was based on research conducted by both

Figure 1

	Recommended Items	Prohibited Items
Beverages	Fresh juices (carrot, chamomile, other herb teas)	Alcohol, cocoa, coffee, milk, soft drinks
Bread	Whole grain breads	no white, enriched breads
Cereals	Whole grain cereals	refined, bleached flour
Dessert	fresh fruit: 3 per day	custards, pastries, puddings, ice creams
Eggs	eggs: only egg substitutes	in any form
Fat	olive oil, butter, sesame oil	shortening, margarine, saturated oils, fats
Fruit	fresh fruit only	canned fruits
Juices	fresh juices only	canned juices, artificially flavored
Meat	none	no pork, fat, fried, smoked meat, sausage; chicken, turkey, or other poultry products
Dairy	raw butter, whipping cream, soy milk, nut milk and seed milks	whole milk, all cheeses
Nuts	fresh, raw nuts, almonds, cashews	roasted, salted nuts and peanuts
Potatoes	baked, boiled potatoes	French fries, chips
Seasoning	chives, garlic, onion, parsley, sage, thyme, sea salt, kelp, sesame salt etc.	hot spices, pepper, sodium salt
Soups	homemade vegetable soups; barley, millet, brown or wild rice	all canned soups, dehydrated soups. No fat stock
Vegetables	raw, freshly cooked vegetables	sprayed, canned or frozen

LIVINGSTON CLINIC DIET

BREAKFAST

8-oz. glass carrot juice containing 1/4 avocado
Basic millet with Nut Cream
Whole grain toast, if desired
Violet leaf tea; supplements as prescribed

LUNCH

Grated carrot with Garden Salad Supreme, horseradish dressing
Black bean soup
Curried Vegetables
Vegetable snack: choice of squash, okra, zucchini, celery, carrots, turnip, and parsnip (raw)
Whole grain bread and butter
Strawberry leaf tea
Supplements as prescribed

DINNER

Garden Salad Supreme
Cream of mushroom soup
Spaghetti squash
Whole grain bread and butter
Peppermint leaf tea
Supplements as prescribed

Figure 2
Foods Containing Abscisic Acid

Fruits	*Vegetables*
mangoes	pea shoots
grapes	lima beans
avocados	potatoes
pears	dwarf peas
oranges with the white underpeel and pulp	sweet potatoes
	asparagus
apples, whole with the seeds	tomatoes
strawberries	onions
	spinach

Fruit blossoms and leaves as tea	*Root vegetables*
peach flowers	All root vegetables—especially carrots
strawberry leaves	
cherry flowers	
apple blossoms	

Leafy vegetables	*Seeds and nuts*
Mature greens	

Source: The Livingston Foundation Medical Center

Livingston and Jackson, which subsequently appeared in several peer review journals.[17]

Patients are urged to eat fruits and vegetables believed to have high amounts of a substance known as *abscisic acid* (see Figure 2). Abscisic acid is a component of vitamin-A related compounds that have been shown to retard the growth of cancer.[18]

Other Scientists Experimenting With Bacterial Vaccines

In 1970, scientists working at the former Institute for Cancer Research in Philadelphia claimed to slow down or prevent the spread of tumors in mice by using a vaccine similar to Livingston's.[19] In another study, Dr. Florence Seibert, a well-known authority on tuberculosis, successfully immunized mice against developing cancer by also using a bacterial vaccine.[20]

In 1972, fifty patients with either "advanced" or "far advanced" cancer were given Livingston's vaccine by a number of independent physicians.[21] While these patients had little hope of a cure, ten had "improved." In addition three seriously ill patients survived for "eight months or longer" after receiving the treatment.[22]

Several years later, French researchers credited a bacterially made vaccine with improving the status of patients suffering from advanced lung cancer. In a five-year clinical study conducted at the Hôpital Saint-Antoine in Paris, the investigators affirmed that their patients enjoyed a better quality of life than those not receiving the vaccine and insisted that their treatment was superior to standard therapies.[23]

Livingston Clinic Success Rate

In 1982, Livingston and her colleagues announced an "82 percent" rate of cure or remission for most forms of cancer via their methods.[24] An independent statistician reportedly calculated this number by the random selection of one hundred patients on file at the Livingston Clinic.

The patients were also reviewed by physicians at the clinic before and after therapy. In all cases, pathology and other medical reports were said to have been required before a pronouncement of "cure" could be made. However, according to the ACS, Livingston's 82 percent cure claim has no basis in scientific fact. Critics point out that the "cured" patients were only required to be without symptoms for one year instead of the official five years before they were considered cured. Moreover, scientific controls were not used as a means of comparing these patients with others in a scientifically designed format. Livingston's therapy is thus considered "unproven" and people are urged not to be treated by it.

American Cancer Society Disputes the Existence of the Cancer Germ

According to both the ACS and the National Cancer Institute (NCI), cancer is not caused by an infectious germ. However, mainstream scientists do believe that viruses, organisms much smaller and different than bacteria, may possibly play a role in causing certain cancers of the throat, cervix, lymphatic system, and liver.[25]

Interestingly, a number of studies that were conducted between 1963 and 1974 as part of an NCI-sponsored investigation have lent some support for the germ theory of cancer—despite the official position against it.[26] For example, NCI researchers reported in 1966 that "the evidence... suggests an association between (a tuberculosis-like germ) and acute leukemia."[27] In another study which appeared in *Annals of the New York Academy of Sciences*, investigators concluded that because they were able to repeatedly isolate "latent [tuberculosis-like germs] from mice" with cancer, the importance of this association should be emphasized.[28]

Shortly before the NCI-sponsored cancer-germ investigation ended, researchers summed up the project as follows:[29]

These studies open very interesting problems; considering the variety and the discrepancies of the results obtained by various [scientists], it seems to us suitable to remain in a waiting position [regarding definite conclusions].

While the NCI largely discounts any of its own favorable reports on a cancer-causing germ, a number of research studies conducted *after* 1974 suggests a correlation between infectious germs and cancer. However, the nature of this correlation still remains a matter of dispute.

Possible Errors in Livingston's Research

Virginia Livingston long maintained that *Progenitor cryptocides* is a tuberculosis-like germ. But independent studies showed that she may have been confusing *Progenitor* with other, more ordinary germs not linked with cancer in any way. According to Dr. Alva H. Johnson, a professor of microbiology at the University of Eastern Virginia Medical School, Livingston's primary error may have been that she failed to conduct follow-up studies to verify her earlier claims.[30]

Dr. Johnson explains that early in Livingston's research, she used the blood of cancer patients to study her alleged cancer germ. Later, when Livingston began using bacteria cultures from the *urine* of patients in order to prepare autogenous vaccines, she assumed that the *Progenitor* organism could also be found in urine; however, when these urine cultures were examined by independent researchers, no evidence of *Progenitor cryptocides* was found.[31]

Dr. Johnson says that this dilemma does not necessarily refute Livingston's theories but only adds to the controversy surrounding them and the urgent need for renewed research.[32]

Credit Attributed to Livingston

In 1974, Livingston made a discovery that some scientists now believe might help solve the enduring puzzle of how cancer cells grow unchecked by the body's immune system. Livingston's discovery involves a growth hormone known as *HCG*.[33] HCG occurs in high concentrations during pregnancy, and it is the same chemical that triggers a positive response in home pregnancy tests.[34, 35]

Livingston theorized that, because the human fetus is a "foreign" protein, it is susceptible to rejection by its mother's immune system. The function of HCG, according to Livingston, is to "surround" the placenta and protect the fetus from its mother's antibodies. Similarly, cancer cells—like the growing fetus—also develop a protective HCG coat which helps them fend off antibodies as well; this is how malignant tumors can grow without facing any substantial resistance from the immune system, according to Livingston.

Livingston also believed that, since cancer bacteria help tumors manufacture their supply of HCG, vaccines such as hers that kill these bacteria would also kill cancer cells. She emphasized that treatments such as radiation, surgery, or chemotherapy, which do not reverse the HCG problem, will never effectively eradicate the cancer.

Of all that Livingston has claimed, her concepts involving HCG have received the strongest support. For example, in 1976, independent scientists verified that bacteria are, in fact, capable of secreting HCG.[36] In addition, a series of experiments has shown that cancer cells produce the hormone.[37, 38]

Livingston's theory that HCG protects both cancer cells and the human fetus has also received the support of numerous investigators who have published their findings in scientific journals such as *Nature* and the *Journal of Experimental Medicine*.[39, 40]

Despite the official stance against most of Livingston's theories, scientists are now studying the potentially significant role of HCG vaccines in cancer treatment.[41]

The Livingston clinic still treats a number of patients yearly. Autogenous vaccines are not being used, but BCG (a well known immunizing agent made from tuberculosis germs), vitamins, minerals, diet treatments, and antibiotics are offered. The estimated cost of treatment at the clinic is $5,500.

While the ACS still officially disputes the Livingston therapy and considers it "unproven," a recent study conducted by the *New England Journal of Medicine (NEJM)* found this treatment as effective as conventional methods when used on terminal cancer patients with little hope for a cure.[42] However, the cornerstone of Livingston's original therapy—autogenous vaccines—was not examined because the Public Health Service and other agencies in California had prohibited their use prior to the *NEJM's* report.[43] The *NEJM* admitted that its own conclusions were "limited" and recognized the necessity of conducting further trials involving patients with some hope for a cure.[44]

Overall, Livingston's concept of treating cancer with bacterial vaccines has received some recent support. In a recent trial conducted at the University of West Virginia, physicians announced that BCG vaccine was proving successful in the treatment of bladder cancer.[45] In an article appearing in the *New York Times*,[46] this vaccine was said to have:

> emerged as an effective, if unlikely weapon against certain bladder cancers that might otherwise require surgery...when

instilled into cancerous bladders...a weakened strain of [tuber-culin-germs] produced a localized tuberculosis infection that seemed to bolster the tumor-fighting ability of the patient's immune system, causing cancers to melt away.

According to Dr. Kevin Pranikoff, a urologist from the State University of New York, the vaccine "is far superior to anything we have and less expensive. I will be using it a lot in the future."[47] Dr. Alva Johnson agrees that bacterial-vaccines may be a "superior" method for treating cancer.[48]

Finally, the actual role of bacteria in cancer, while officially disputed, continues to be explored by a small number of research scientists. In some cases, a correlation has been noted and documented in peer-approved review journals.

For further information contact:

The Livingston Foundation Medical Center
3232 Duke Street
San Diego, CA 92110
(619) 224-3515

FOUR

Hydrazine Sulfate

In 1968, a Syracuse, New York, physician named Joseph Gold wrote a paper proposing a new way to deal with the cancer problem.

Dr. Gold hypothesized that most cancer deaths result from cachexia (k∂-kek'sē∂)—the devastating process whereby cancer patients experience severe malnutrition and weight loss. Based on this theory, Gold searched for a substance that could reverse the wasting syndrome. After some investigation, he concluded that hydrazine sulfate, an inexpensive chemical that is used industrially and commercially, might work.

After developing a method to purify the drug, Gold began testing it on animals and then later published papers on his research. In these papers, Gold reported that hydrazine was, unlike other cancer drugs, relatively safe and nontoxic. Even more impressive, the drug seemed to work by correcting faulty metabolism in the body rather than by poisoning large numbers of cells as chemotherapy agents do; in this sense, hydrazine was potentially the first in a new class of anticancer drugs designed to work with and not against the body.

One physician who had heard of Gold's research tried hydrazine on a desperately ill patient and reported good results. After a number of other cancer patients began taking the drug and reporting similar benefits, hydrazine began to receive considerable media attention.

In 1973, Sloan-Kettering Cancer Center agreed to test hydrazine sulfate on a small group of patients. But Sloan-Kettering doctors failed to observe any positive results and concluded the drug was without merit. Because of this negative finding, the American Cancer Society (ACS) placed hydrazine sulfate on its *Unproven Therapies List.*

Gold immediately protested that Sloan-Kettering had not involved him in its study and had also failed to use the proper doses of hydrazine recommended by him. To counter what he claimed was a biased report, Gold published his own paper on a hydrazine trial involving eighty-four patients. In this trial, the majority of patients experienced "subjective improvements" such as weight gain, improved appetite, and a lessening of pain. Some patients also experienced "objective improvements" such as shrinking of tumors.[1]

After a number of clinical studies in the United States confirmed the therapeutic action of hydrazine, it was vindicated as an effective anticancer drug. The drug has since been removed from the *Unproven Therapies List.* Still, controversy remains and this treatment has not been endorsed for general use.

Currently, patients may apply for hydrazine sulfate through their physician.

Dr. Gold's Background

The physician received his medical degree from Upstate Medical Center of the State University of New York in 1956.[2]

After graduation, Gold served as a U.S. Air Force medical research physician for the Mercury astronaut program. He was involved in the exclusive preparation of astronaut trainees and certified John Glenn fit for lift-off.[3] After returning to Syracuse and entering full-time medical practice, Dr. Gold became extensively involved in cancer research.

The physician has authored more than a dozen scientific papers on cancer and related treatment; his papers have appeared in a number of peer-review journals, including *Nutrition and Cancer*, *Oncology*, and *Annals of the New York Academy of Sciences.*[4]

The Rationale for Using Hydrazine Sulfate

Because cachexia is considered the foremost contributor to patient mortality from cancer,[5, 6] Dr. Gold reasoned that by reversing this wasting syndrome, cancer itself could be inhibited or even stopped.

To better understand how cachexia develops, Gold studied the pioneering work of Nobel-prize winning scientist Otto Warburg. In the 1930s, Warburg conducted a series of experiments that he believed unraveled a major piece of the cancer puzzle (see also chapter 2).

According to Warburg, cancer cells thrive in an environment having little or no oxygen. Unlike healthy cells which derive their energy from glucose (blood sugar) and oxygen, cancer cells draw their energy by *fermenting* glucose in what is largely an "airless" reaction. This "fermentation" process causes a number of waste products to form in the body, one of which is lactic acid.[7] Since lactic acid serves no useful purpose, the liver converts it back into usable glucose.

Gold used Warburg's controversial theory as a starting point and then advanced his own concept of how cachexia develops. He reasoned that cancer cells only partially burn up glucose. However, because their energy requirements for glucose are so high, the constant recycling of lactic acid back into sugar provides cancer cells with a virtually unlimited source of energy while, at the same time, draining the body's normal energy reserves.

Gold believed that if a way could be found to block the reconversion of lactic acid into glucose, then the cancer cell would be robbed of its valuable fuel supply and the devastating cachexia process might be reversed. In essence, the "sick relationship" (as Gold described it) between cancer and the liver would be interrupted.

How Hydrazine was Discovered

Dr. Gold tested a variety of chemical agents that might block the lactic-acid/glucose cycle. Finally, he discovered a biochemist's report identifying hydrazine sulfate as a drug that could perform this function.[8]

In its original form, hydrazine is used as a chemical reducing agent, antioxidant, and jet fuel. But Gold subjected it to a purification process and tested very small amounts on animals. After testing showed no major side effects, Gold's next step was to conduct human trials.

Hydrazine Sulfate's Results on People

Dr. Gold treated about one hundred patients in the early 1970s. In addition, Russian doctors were actively testing hydrazine on a larger scale. In these early trials, hydrazine reversed the "wasting" process in up to 70 percent of the patients.[9] In addition, 41 percent of the patients reportedly experienced a cessation of tumor growth.[10]

Shortly afterward, officials at Sloan-Kettering expressed an interest in studying hydrazine.

The Sloan-Kettering Trial

After treating twenty-nine patients with hydrazine sulfate, Sloan-Kettering researcher Dr. Manuel Ochoa reported the following results:

1. None of the patients responded positively.
2. Nearly 50 percent of the patients developed symptoms of nerve damage.

Based on Dr. Ochoa's results, Sloan-Kettering concluded that hydrazine sulfate was not effective in the treatment of human cancer and might even prove harmful.[11]

Dr. Gold found a number of faults in the study. He objected that patients were never given the correct doses of hydrazine which he had carefully formulated; nerve damage only occurred when patients were given too much of the drug; and Sloan-Kettering did not mention that subjective improvements occurred in a number of patients.[12] In addition, Gold pointed out that hydrazine sulfate shows fewer positive effects when used on a short-term basis as in the Sloan-Kettering trial.

After the failed trial, Dr. Gold published the results of his own refutational study in the medical journal *Oncology*. A number of studies conducted by Russian scientists also contradicted the Sloan-Kettering findings.

The Russian Hydrazine Trials

During the 1970s, Russian scientists were taking a great deal of interest in hydrazine and like Gold, claimed significant results in animal and human studies.[13, 14]

In what is considered the largest and lengthiest trial of its kind, hydrazine sulfate was administered to a total of 740 Russian patients suffering from "widespread...metastatic" tumors for an eight-year period.[15] Among the various cancers treated were those of the lung, stomach, colon, breast, and cervix. As a rule, lung and stomach malignancies are among the least treatable forms of cancer.[16]

The Russian patients were meticulously screened to fulfill certain testing criteria. For example, all the patients were terminal and had exhausted all other conventional modes of therapy; drug dosing was designed strictly according to Dr. Gold's recommendations; use of medications which might interfere with the study results were prohibited and patients were to have received no other cancer treatments for at least six weeks prior to the trial.

While the researchers emphasized that that their patients were "all . . . in the terminal phase of the disease"[17] "stabilization" of cancer was still noted in 40 percent. Moreover, a number of subjective responses not usually seen with other therapies was reported. For example, "pronounced" improvements were noted in appetite and strength levels; respiratory problems, fluid buildup, and fever were reduced; and a "complete elimination of pain" was observed frequently.[18] In several instances of severely debilitating bone cancer, hydrazine had such a profound effect that patients could move about without help for the first time in the course of their illness.[19]

In a number of cases, an uplift in mood—even to the point of "giddiness" and euphoria—was listed as a side effect. A few cases of possible nerve damage were noted, but these resulted from "prolonged" and "uninterrupted" use of hydrazine. The Russians found that by interrupting treatment for specified periods, they could administer hydrazine safely and without adverse effects for as long as ten years.[20]

Shortly after the Russians submitted a paper on their hydrazine results to the 7th Annual Meeting of the American Association for Cancer Research in 1979,[21] the ACS removed hydrazine sulfate from its *Unproven Therapies List.*

Renewed Interest Among Orthodox Researchers

In 1984, scientists at University of California at Los Angeles (UCLA) began a series of clinically controlled studies to reevaluate hydrazine sulfate. The senior investigator in charge of these studies was Rowan Chlebowski, a physician/researcher affiliated with the UCLA School of Medicine and the Clinical Research Center, Harbor-

UCLA Medical Center. Dr. Chlebowski spearheaded four studies on hydrazine lasting through 1990.

The first of the studies was a "prospective, double-blind" trial designed to examine hydrazine's effect on the body's metabolism.[22] One group of patients received the drug and the other group, a placebo. Neither the researchers nor the patients knew who received the actual drug, and thus any chance of bias was eliminated.

After thirty days of treatment, hydrazine sulfate was found to cause statistically significant improvement in the way in which patients were able to use blood sugar.[23] In addition, the majority of these patients gained weight and experienced few side effects.

The second study was launched in 1985. Fifty-eight terminally ill patients, most of whom suffered from lung cancer, were also observed in a blind study. One month after treatment began, Dr. Chlebowski and his colleagues reported that 78 percent of the patients taking hydrazine maintained or increased their weight versus 38 percent in the placebo group.[24]

In the third study, hydrazine was tested on yet a larger group of 101 cancer patients. After comparing the treated with the placebo group, Chlebowski found that 83 percent of the hydrazine patients gained or maintained their weight against 53 percent of the controls; 63 percent enjoyed better appetite against only 25 percent, and calorie intake increased in the hydrazine group by 14 percent.[25]

The fourth and final hydrazine trial was among the most important performed at UCLA. In this landmark study, all participating patients were terminally ill and suffering from the end-stages of lung cancer. The prognosis of these patients was bleak and the only treatment available to them—aggressive chemotherapy—could be expected to increase survival by only several months.[26]

Sixty-five of the patients were paired into two groups. Approximately half received hydrazine and a combination of conventional cancer drugs; the other half, only the cancer drugs and a placebo. After the courses of treatment were evaluated, the hydrazine sulfate group showed significantly better improvement than the placebo group.[27]

Hydrazine's greatest impact was seen in patients who were not bedridden and could move about. In this group, the drug "significantly prolonged" life—328 days against only 209 days for the controls.

After one year of treatment, 42 percent of the hydrazine patients were alive against 18 percent of the placebo-taking patients.[28] Of equal significance, hydrazine was found to help people maintain levels of a blood protein known as albumin; this effect is crucial because albumin loss in cancer patients is associated with shorter survival time and can even serve as a yardstick to determine how long people will live.[29]

The researchers concluded that hydrazine sulfate resulted in overall greater survival rates compared with other therapies available for the patients in their study group. They also emphasized that treatment strategies which improve the body's metabolism—as hydrazine does—"represents a fundamentally new direction for clinical cancer management."[30]

The UCLA conclusions were further supported by British scientists in 1987. Reporting in the medical journal *Lancet*, the scientists found that hydrazine-treated patients had a greater ability to retain proteins, maintain body weight and preserve levels of albumin. The investigators concluded that "an important predictor of 2-year survival in lung cancer patients is the maintenance of serum albumin... so the metabolic changes induced by the hydrazine group may prove clinically beneficial."[31]

National Cancer Institute Researchers Contradict the UCLA Findings

In 1991, the NCI completed a twenty-month trial on 291 patients receiving hydrazine sulfate at the Scripps Clinic in San Diego.

Dr. Michael Kosty, the trial director, reported that hydrazine sulfate did not prolong the lives of cancer patients nor did it improve appetite or result in weight gain. Worse, it might even have caused nerve damage in a number of the patients. Kosty disputed Chlebowski's findings, calling the four UCLA studies "meaningless."[32]

An Investigative Reporter Uncovers Serious Discrepancies in the Kosty Study

Jeff Kamen, a medical reporter, became a leading hydrazine activist after his mother—suffering from cancer and given only days to live—

survived an additional four months on hydrazine therapy. Kamen believes his mother would have fared better had doctors not discontinued her treatment.[33]

In a 1992 interview, Dr. Maxwell Gordon, a former Bristol-Myers vice president and onetime proponent of hydrazine, told Kamen that after learning of Dr. Kosty's plans to test hydrazine, he phoned the researcher and cautioned him about the use of extraneous drugs, medications, or alcohol in the trial patients; these substances are believed to totally negate any of hydrazine's positive effects. Although Gordon "emphasized the importance of [the drug] exclusions" he was "at a loss" to explain why they did not follow his recommendations. Oddly, Dr. Kosty admitted to Kamen that "no commitments to include [or] exclude specific medications" were ever made.[34] Based on this factor, Kamen argues that the Kosty trial "demonstrates nothing."

Further underscoring the possible flaws in Kosty's study, Kamen points to a separately planned hydrazine trial at the Mayo Clinic in which researchers will prohibit the extraneous use of any substance or drug which might bias their final results.

Despite the number of statistically favorable reports on hydrazine sulfate, a recent multi-institutional trial sponsored by the NCI claims to dispute the drug's value. But critics argue that the NCI study did not follow its originally designed protocol.

According to Jeff Kamen, the intended purpose of the NCI's most recent study was to evaluate hydrazine on early-stage cancer patients (all other trials have involved terminally-ill individuals). In contradiction of its own protocol, however, the patients all suffered from "late-stage" cancers.[35] For this reason, Kamen—who is at the forefront of a movement to legitimize and distribute hydrazine on a national scale—calls the NCI study "superfluous."

Kamen and other critics believe there are inherent biases against hydrazine sulfate beyond the realm of pure science. They point to examples of vested interests subverting hydrazine because of the drug's poor profit potential and also to unfair press coverage perpetrated by influential people.

For example, a highly regarded John Hopkins cancer physician criticized the UCLA studies as unreliable because Chlebowski's study group was too small to reach any meaningful conclusions. However, the UCLA researchers carefully organized their trial to meet "its prospectively determined target size of 60 patients" and had, by all accounts, fulfilled the necessary conditions demanded by protocol.[36] But even if trial size had been a problem, very little notice had been given the favorable Soviet trials, which involved far greater populations of patients than any one of the UCLA, Scripps, or NCI studies. Further, while orthodox critics were quick to seize on such technical issues as patient size in the favorable Chlebowski studies, they seemed not to notice such glaring problems as the possible biasing of secondary drugs in the Kosty study—by far a more significant concern.

One factor which appears to split consensus over hydrazine involves the conflicting goals sought after by researchers. Traditionally, more weight is given to "objective" rather than "subjective" measurements of progress against cancer. As a consequence, researchers are primarily concerned with the visible effects drugs have on killing cancer cells, rather than on how better people feel or function.

In this regard, hydrazine sulfate has the paradoxical quality of showing either beneficial effects against cancer, or few effects—depending on which perspective it is viewed from. Chlebowski believes this factor explains[37] why

> [hydrazine] trials which used subjective therapeutic endpoints have largely reported positive results, whereas small trials of hydrazine... where reduction in tumor size was used as [a] therapeutic endpoint, have reported little benefit.

Proponents of hydrazine sulfate therapy admit that it does not directly kill tumors but can raise crucial parameters of health which, in turn, may allow people to manage their illnesses better. In this regard, if people eat more, take less pain medication, gain weight, and experience less albumin loss, these effects are tangible and can thus be considered objective measurements of benefit.

Interestingly, hydrazine's possible actions against tumor growth have not been ruled out; a number of cancer remissions have been reported.

At this time, hydrazine sulfate is not being viewed as a single cancer treatment but may prove a beneficial adjunct to other therapies—traditional or alternative. While lung cancers have been the most studied cases in America involving the drug, other types of malignancies have shown benefit.

For further information contact:

Dr. Joseph Gold
Syracuse Cancer Research Institute
600 East Genesee Street
Syracuse, NY 13202
(315) 472-6616

FIVE

Immuno-Augmentative Therapy

During the 1950s, two New York University zoology students isolated a *tumor factor* from fruit flies and mice that could cause cancer in healthy animals. After completing their postgraduate studies, Lawrence Burton and Frank Friedman joined the cancer research wing of St. Vincent's Hospital in Manhattan and embarked on a quest for the protein which could block the tumor-causing factor.

In 1959, the two scientists announced that they had, in fact, succeeded in isolating a "tumor-inhibiting factor." Remarkably, when this protein was injected into cancer-stricken mice, tumors would simply shrivel up and die—not in days or weeks but in a matter of *hours* according to eyewitness reports. Later, the researchers began to develop methods to apply their findings to human cancers.

In 1974, Burton and Friedman left St. Vincent's and established a clinic in Great Neck, New York. A purified version of tumor-inhibiting factor was then used to treat human cancer patients with incurable malignancies. This treatment was said to cure 15 percent of the patients.

Attempts to conduct a clinical study of the tumor-inhibiting factor never came to fruition after negotiations between Burton and federal cancer agencies collapsed. The National Cancer Institute (NCI) maintained that it tried to launch a trial but blamed Burton and Friedman for being uncooperative and unwilling to share information.

The two scientists complained that they were unable to receive funding, were stymied from publishing their controversial work, and were eventually reprimanded for manufacturing an illegal serum. According to Burton, this series of events forced him to leave the country and establish a cancer clinic in Freeport, Grand Bahamas, in 1977.

A number of further attempts were made by federal agencies to test Burton's serum. But the scientist—often described as secretive and paranoid—was wary of antagonism toward him by some quarters of organized medicine and was said to be unyielding in the negotiations. Then in 1985, the Burton controversy suddenly exploded into a major scandal when vials of his serum were alleged to have AIDS contamination. The clinic was immediately shut down, and hundreds of angered patients, convinced that Burton's therapy was their only hope, called for a Congressional investigation. The patients found an ally in New York Congressman Guy Molinari, who launched a probe on their behalf. After the charges against Burton were found to be exaggerated, and "untruths" on the part of various federal agencies were revealed, the clinic reopened less than a year after its shutdown.

Several years after the AIDS scare, Burton's controversial method (which later came to be known as "Immuno-Augmentative Therapy" or IAT) was investigated by a team of researchers at the University of Pennsylvania. While the team's initial prepublished report showed positive results from IAT, the final revision claims to offer no favorable conclusions. This report has been harshly criticized for a number of reasons.

Burton died in 1993, but patients are still being treated at his clinic under the supervision of Dr. Robert Clement.

Therapy in the Bahamas normally lasts from 6 to 8 weeks and is dependent on the severity of a person's illness. After treatment, injections are continued at home and these may last for weeks or months. Afterward, periodic checkups to help reevaluate immunity are scheduled and performed at the clinic. IAT costs $5,000 for the first four weeks and $500 for each additional week thereafter. Injections used by patients at home are $50 weekly.[1]

At this time, IAT remains on the list of unproven cancer remedies of the American Cancer Society (ACS).

Lawrence Burton and his Qualifications in Human Cancer Treatment

Born in New York City in 1926, Lawrence Burton received a B.S. degree from Brooklyn College, an M.S. from New York University and a doctorate in zoology from the California Institute of Technology.[2] While a graduate student at Cal Tech, Burton concentrated on genetics, immunobiology, and cancer causation in animals and humans as his major fields of study.[3]

As a professional, Burton was a Research Associate in Pathology, Associate in Oncology, Senior Investigator, and Senior Oncologist at St. Vincent's Hospital in Manhattan. He also taught genetics and bacteriology at New York University. The scientist's peer-review articles have appeared in *Transactions of the New York Academy of Sciences*, *Cancer Research*, and *Science*.[4]

Dr. Burton's Theory on the Cause of Cancer

Many immunologists believe that the human body has a capability for recognizing and destroying cancer cells. However, scientists are not precisely sure why this capability is not normally unleashed in cancer patients. Burton believed he found an answer to the puzzle. The scientist hypothesized that human beings possess a series of proteins or "factors" that are capable of regulating cancer growth. These protein factors consist of the following four components:

1. Tumor antibody
2. Tumor complement factor
3. Blocking protein factor
4. Deblocking protein factor

Burton's view was that a healthy immune system could detect tumor "markers" (also called "tumor complement") and then zero in on cancer cells accordingly. There is, however, a downside to this scenario. According to Burton, if malignant cells are destroyed too rapidly, the liver can become overwhelmed by dying masses of malignant tissue, and potentially serious complications could then result. (Interestingly, this theory is similar to the one advanced by Dr. Max Gerson, chapter 2). As a safeguard, nature provided human beings with a blood protein known as "blocking factor," and its purpose is to regulate the rate of cancer-cell destruction.

Burton believed that in sick people, there is actually too much blocking factor; this imbalance causes the immune system to *over-regulate* cancer-killing antibodies. In essence, an excess of blocking factor is what allows cancer cells to grow.

The crux of Burton's treatment strategy lies in another factor which he named *deblocking protein*; by increasing the levels of this protein in sick people, Burton believed that their antibodies could be reactivated to systematically destroy cancer cells.

How Immuno-Augmentative Therapy Is Believed to Work

The aim of IAT is to reestablish and put into balance individual levels of the four protein factors. If, for example, a patient is found to have too much blocking protein but not enough deblocker, the correct amounts (or "titers") of deblockers are administered.

To determine whether an excess or deficiency of one of the factors exists in cancer patients, blood levels are analyzed once or twice daily. This information is then submitted into a computer and an appropriate treatment strategy is formulated.

How the Burton Serum Is Made

Healthy donors are used to make tumor antibodies and deblocking factor because these proteins are believed lacking in people with cancer. Conversely, tumor complement is taken from the cancer patient, because healthy people would not be likely to have large amounts of cancer proteins in their bodies.

The Burton Clinic's Rate of Success

During the three years that Burton and Friedman treated patients in Great Neck, they claimed about a 15 percent rate of remission; the vast majority of their patients were considered terminally ill with no hope of recovery.[5] A later follow-up of the first 277 patients treated in the Bahamas was said to show an 18 percent rate of remission.[6] These patients had all exhausted the benefits of conventional medicine and were considered untreatable. If these remission rates are correct, they would exceed the expected conventional cure rates, estimated at about 1 percent for similar categories of cancer.[7]

While the ACS disputes the curative potential of IAT, independent clinicians and a large number of patients have reported positive results.

Independent Reports on IAT

In the 1970s, Dr. John Beaty, a medical doctor affiliated with Greenwich Hospital in Connecticut, referred twenty "far advanced" cancer patients to the Bahamas for treatment. In Beaty's estimation, half experienced verifiable tumor regression.[8] Beaty stated that his patients owed their "very survival" to Burton and insisted that the scientist had found a "breakthrough" in cancer research.[9] Overall, the Greenwich physician testified that he had "seen many, many patients who have benefited from Dr. Burton's therapy."[10]

The recent testimony of a New Jersey surgeon may shed more light on the potential effectiveness of IAT. During sworn testimony before Congressman Guy Molinari in 1986, Dr. Phillip Kunderman expressed "amazement" at the results he said were being achieved by IAT.

A graduate of Cornell Medical School and a board certified surgeon, Dr. Kunderman had served as past president of the New Jersey chapter's American College of Surgeons. He was also chief of surgery and chief of thoracic surgery at five New Jersey hospitals. As a matter of record, Dr. Kunderman stated that he had "tremendous experience with cancer," having treated "pretty much all of the chest cancer that occurred in the Central New Jersey area."[11]

After developing metastatic cancer of the prostate for which there was no effective cure, Kunderman traveled to the Bahamas and investigated Burton's therapy for himself. During his review, Kunderman became especially interested in the treatment results for a rare form of asbestos-related cancer known as mesothelioma—a particularly deadly malignancy that attacks the lining of the lungs. Located near a major asbestos producer in New Jersey, Dr. Kunderman had seen firsthand many cases of mesothelioma which he said showed a "horrendously poor" prognosis.[12]

After carefully reviewing the IAT clinic's records and pathology reports, Kunderman "marveled" that a number of mesothelioma patients were actually surviving for many years and living normal lives. The New Jersey surgeon then began his own course of treatment and remained alive and well six years after his terminal prognosis.[13]

Kunderman, who remarked that he "had never encountered" treatment results like Burton's, told Congressman Molinari:

> I know of carcinoma of the pancreas which, in my experience, was such a lethal, terrible carcinoma, with remission for as long as eight or nine years, carcinoma of the larynx, and the [patient has survived at least ten years], and these were such horrible cancers.[14]

The physician concluded that he was "convinced" IAT is "the right approach" in the treatment of advanced cancer according to present-day standards.

Another physician who shared Kunderman's enthusiasm was the former president of the Bahamian Medical Association, Dr. Robert J. Clement. Clement (who now supervises the Burton Clinic), stated that in a five-year time span, 1,500 patients treated with IAT showed "better results than chemotherapy and radiation."[15]

Why IAT Is Not Endorsed by the American Cancer Society

In the absence of appropriate clinical trials, IAT is not considered a proven therapy for cancer despite the "testimonial" evidence offered by "cured" patients. The ACS argues that personal claims are not scientific proof of IAT's worth. Moreover, the claims that have been made are considered highly questionable. For example, in 1981, a number of Burton's patients submitted sworn affidavits to Florida legislators, attesting to the favorable effects of IAT. But the affidavits were issued only two to six months after treatments were started, and this time span does not constitute a scientific measure of success.[16]

According to a physician investigating the claims, two of Burton's patients died before their testimonies were even presented to lawmakers.[17] In one case, a patient's bone cancer—said to have gone into remission—actually worsened. The physician explained that post-treatment bone scans purporting to show no evidence of cancer were negative simply because the bone had been literally destroyed by tumors and thus did not show anything—cancer or otherwise.[18]

Summing up its portrayal of IAT, the ACS quotes a Pompano Beach cancer physician who treated or consulted 15 of Burton's patients. At a press conference, the physician stated that he was impressed with the "tender, loving, care" offered patients by Burton's staff. But he added that his experiences with the 15 patients—14 of whom had died—were "nothing short of disastrous."[19]

Since the majority of patients receive IAT well after their initial diagnosis and the start of conventional treatment, it would be extremely difficult to interpret the "failures" cited by the ACS; by that agency's own standard, cancer therapy should always be instituted at the earliest possible time before disease progression has gone too far.

Why Scientific Trials of IAT Have Not Been Conducted by Government Agencies

Initially, interest in testing IAT was expressed by federal agencies. In 1975, the NCI submitted a formal questionnaire to Dr. Burton as a prerequisite for testing. But according to the Food and Drug Administration (FDA), Burton never adequately answered the questions necessary for securing an IND (Investigation of New Drug), and his application was simply rejected.[20] But Burton told a different story.

During sworn testimony, Burton explained that the FDA's questions were designed to frustrate attempts at a "fair trial." For instance, the FDA asked what outcome IAT would have on cat leukemia; in Burton's estimation, it would have taken years to develop and test IAT on cat-related leukemias and thus the question was not relevant to the issue of human cancer.

Burton also cited moral and ethical imperatives for not cooperating in an NCI trial; the scientist had continually objected against double-blind studies which, in his words, would have allowed "fifty patients" a chance at life and the other fifty controls, a "condemnation to death."[21]

Why Dr. Burton Relocated to the Bahamas

One of Burton's primary motivations for leaving the country was that the medical journals refused to publish his work and were, in effect, "blackballing" him. To support this claim, Burton pointed out that he and Friedman easily published fourteen articles in respected journals between the period 1959 and 1963. But when his concepts became controversial, the articles were no longer being published.

Much has been written about Burton's plight with the medical establishment. Some critics say the scientist was eccentric, suspicious, and paranoid and that he perpetuated antagonism toward his own work through an unwillingness to cooperate with key players in cancer science.

Other observers believe that key events during Burton's career justify his suspicions. One event supporting this contention occurred in the early 1960s. During that time, Burton and Friedman were funded by two prestigious sources: the NCI and the Damon Runyon Memorial Fund for Cancer Research. Their work also attracted the attention of Sloan-Kettering Cancer Center.

Sloan-Kettering dispatched Dr. John J. Harris, one of its senior investigators, to Burton's laboratory. In a later interview, Harris admitted that he was actually sent to St. Vincent's with the objective of "smuggling" back as much information as I could. I didn't go for that, and Friedman, Burton and I published everything that went on. This got disapproval back at the lab."[22]

Later, when Harris collaborated with Burton on a paper, Sloan-Kettering officials were angered because Harris's name was listed last, not first.[23] Shortly afterward, Burton and Friedman lost their funding and Harris was pressured into leaving Sloan-Kettering. This account was verified by Harris's widow in 1979.

Burton claims that after funds were terminated, he found it increasingly difficult to publish his work. For example, a paper submitted to the prestigious *Proceedings of the Society for Experimental Biology and Medicine* was rejected because Burton's terminology was considered too theoretical and lacked conventional familiarity.[24] The journal's editors remarked that they could not tell whether the proteins Burton described consisted of "stinkweed or roses."[25]

Burton labeled this incident one example of a malicious unwillingness to accept his controversial ideas.

Attempts to Launch a Clinical Trial of IAT

Following a favorable *60 Minutes* news report on Burton in 1980,[26] renewed interest in IAT stirred among legislators, who later drafted a bill to limit U.S. import bans on Burton's vaccines.

Two years after the *60 Minutes* presentation, former NCI director Dr. Vincent DeVita contacted Burton with the intent of launching an appropriate clinical trial. But Burton replied with an accusatory letter complaining that DeVita's associates had made slanderous remarks about IAT, calling it a fraud.[27] Burton protested that, under such circumstances, it would be extremely difficult for the NCI to objectively assess his treatment. Shortly afterward, negotiations broke down.

Many observers feel that Burton should have put aside personal animosities and worked with Dr. DeVita and the NCI for the betterment of cancer patients.

Controversy Surrounding the Burton Clinic

In May 1985, 18 vials of IAT serum were submitted by a Burton patient for testing at a Tacoma, Washington, blood bank, and 8 were said to be "borderline or positive" for the AIDS virus.[28] In addition, all 18 vials were "positive" for hepatitis B antigen.[29] Upon repeat testing by the Centers for Disease Control (CDC), 6 of the 18 samples tested positive for AIDS while 13 were positive for hepatitis.[30] Based on these findings, the Burton clinic was immediately shut down and considered a health hazard. Worldwide news organizations then aired stories describing the clinic as unsanitary and actively spreading the deadly AIDS virus. At a gathering of the National Health Fraud Conference, President Reagan's Special Adviser for Consumer Affairs warned that the Burton clinic had been responsible "for at least several hundred cases of AIDS worldwide."[31]

In response to the shutdown, a group of IAT patients—convinced that the AIDS data was inaccurate and largely contrived—formed an organization and demanded a Congressional review. Seven months after the closure, an inquiry conducted by Congressman Guy Molinari substantiated many of the patients' charges and the clinic was allowed to reopen.[32]

Revelation of the IATPA Investigation

The IATPA (an abbreviation for "Immuno-Augmentative Therapy Patients Association") was primarily interested in resolving the AIDS controversy because most members felt their lives to be in jeopardy— not from AIDS, but from a discontinuance of Burton's treatment.

After the Molinari investigation, previously unpublicized revelations came to light which contradicted the government's stance against Burton. According to the IATPA, these revelations have been documented and were derived from the following sources:

—The Freedom of Information Act
—Tape-recorded telephone conversations
—Data obtained from IAT patient records
—Congressional records

In an affidavit procured through the Freedom of Information Act, IATPA investigators found that while some of the allegedly tainted serum samples were initially believed to be "marginally or slightly positive" for AIDS antibodies via the standardized ELISA blood screen, follow-up testing with the more accurate Western-blot test showed none to be positive and all to be negative.[33] ELISA tests are considered highly accurate in determining whether antibodies to the AIDS virus are actually in blood samples but occasionally yield* positive responses even when samples are negative.[34]

Interestingly, when the Centers for Disease Control (CDC) was notified of the problem, "no effort" was made to impound supplies of Burton's serum at their source, nor to determine the distribution of the serum—an unusual response if there had indeed been an outbreak. In an interview conducted by the nutritionist and health writer Gary Null, the patient who brought vials of IAT serum into Tacoma for testing claims that she was never asked to provide names of patients to whom the vials belonged nor was any history taken on the origin and transport of the vials.[35]

It has never been established precisely *how* the AIDS virus was cultured from Burton's serum; screening procedures available at the time were generally limited to testing human blood and not the type of "processed serum" made by Burton. According to a leading researcher at the University of California at Los Angeles (UCLA), the dilemma of how to effectively screen serum products for AIDS was (in 1985) as yet, an unsolved "mystery."[36] CDC scientist Dr. Harold Jaffe added that "the tests [for AIDS antibodies] were not designed to be used on whatever is in this material [Burton's serum]."[37] Based on

---

*This type of inaccurate response is known as a "false positive" test.

these and other ambiguities, Dr. Gregory Curt (one of the investigators who reported isolating HIV from the Burton samples) announced: "we can't say [the Tacoma samples result]...is a positive test."[38]

In retrospect, there is evidence that the CDC was, in reality, not worried about an AIDS "outbreak." For example, in a taped telephone conversation, a government official commented that:

> One out of nine vials had been found to contain the virus. It is not unusual to find AIDS virus in blood or blood products. If you look for it, you're probably going to find it when you look at a number of samples like that [i.e., the Burton samples].[39]

Indeed, national AIDS screening during the four-week period April through May 1985 revealed some shocking findings. Medical investigator Robert G. Houston discovered that 5,313 units of blood tested positive for AIDS at 131 blood banks throughout the United States; upon repeat testing, only 25 percent were considered true positives.[40] In comparison, only one of the Burton samples had been documented as being AIDS positive.

Whatever the true quantity of possible contamination in the Burton serum, data from 1985 has revealed that in all probability, the *entire* United States supply of immune globulin (a blood protein the origin of which is similar to that of Burton's blood fractions) was positive for AIDS antibodies.[41] According to a physician who had become concerned about this fact, the CDC told him that "all the current supply [of immune globulin] available in the United States is, indeed, known to be positive for the [AIDS] antibody."[42] Significantly, the presence of AIDS antibodies in properly sterilized medical products does not pose a health hazard if all traces of the AIDS virus have been killed. People who receive such products, however, may still test "positive" for AIDS—without actually being infected—because their immune systems have become sensitized to the inactivated viral proteins.

Shortly after the AIDS controversy at the Burton Clinic, fifty-four IAT patients were voluntarily screened and all tested negative.[43] As of this writing, no one receiving Immuno-Augmentative therapy has been known to develop AIDS nor test positive for the actual virus. There have been accounts, however, of people contracting hepatitis through IAT products. In 1984, for example, *The New England Journal of Medicine* reported that one patient came down with IAT-related hepatitis.[44] In addition, IATPA officials launched their own investigation in 1985 and found that two patients had contracted the disease in a similar fashion.[45]

The Burton clinic is not unique regarding hepatitis infection. In general, the chance of contracting hepatitis in the United States during the course of medical treatment has been estimated at 3 percent to 10 percent.[46] And despite highly controlled screening procedures, routine tests for hepatitis in blood products are considered less than accurate.[47]

Further, while much emphasis has been placed on hepatitis B found in samples of the Burton serum, researchers have noticed a troublesome upswing in the incidence of hepatitis C infection in recent years throughout the United States. This virus—believed responsible for 90 percent of all hepatitis cases received through processed blood[48]— poses a major health threat, since it has been implicated in liver cancer, cirrhosis, and other life-threatening diseases like its hepatitis B cousin.[49]

For patients receiving serum injections, preventive vaccines for hepatitis are available. These can be supplied by the patient's physician.

Current Clinic Safeguards Against AIDS and Other Infections

Prior to the clinic's closing, the following five methods of sterilization[50] were already in place:

1. Testing of blood products by injecting samples into animals
2. Ultra-filtration
3. Freezing to −178C
4. Ultraviolet light
5. Sedimentation procedures.

During the Molinari investigation, Burton testified that animals were used as a "foolproof" method for screening blood products. IAT serum was also "driven" through special filters said to remove "all known viruses and bacteria." Afterward, batches of serum were placed in an airtight room" and bathed in ultraviolet light each night to insure maximum sterility.[51]

Despite these procedures, an infectious outbreak did occur among clinic patients in 1984 and was caused by a "soil bacterium" known as

Nocardia asteroides. According to the CDC, sixteen patients were infected and all developed abscesses.[52]

Burton explained that the *Nocardia* organism was introduced into his facility via an air conditioning duct connected to the Rand hospital complex; in 1984, the Burton clinic was actually an annex of that hospital. After the 1985 closure, a new clinic was built and was subjected to strict guidelines imposed by Bahamian authorities as a condition for remaining open.[53]

How the Medical Profession Views IAT

The last independent study of IAT was conducted in 1987 by Dr. Barrie Cassileth and colleagues at the University of Pennsylvania. In that study, seventy-nine patients treated by IAT were observed.[54] Forty-eight percent of the patients were said to have a variety of progressive, inoperable cancers.

In the first draft of Cassileth's study,[55] the following results were noted:

—63 percent of the patients were still alive five years after diagnosis; expected survival was less than three years

—33 percent of the patients had an improvement in ambulatory status (i.e., the ability to move about)

—29 percent had improved appetites

Overall, the IAT patients were found to survive 75 percent longer than people using conventional therapies.

After the report was drafted, however, Dr. Cassileth negated most of her favorable study conclusions because of "positive biasing factors." For example, while patients may have indeed improved after receiving Burton's treatment, such factors as "age," "race" and "socio-economic" background were believed to falsely boost the results.[56]

Following are the positive biases cited by Dr. Cassileth and her colleagues:

—Because cancer patients who traveled to the Bahamas for treatment were more likely to be in better physical condition, later "improvements" in mobility were not due to IAT and reflect a "selection bias."

—The age of the IAT patients was, on average, younger than cancer patients treated in the United States; this factor would obviously affect treatment outcomes more positively.

—The IAT patients were all white and of higher social privilege and opportunity.

Criticism of the Positive Biases Argument

A number of flaws have been cited. For example, the notion that people going to the Bahamas for treatment do better because they are more mobile has been contradicted by an unrelated study performed at the Mayo Clinic in Rochester, Minnesota.

All of the seriously ill cancer patients involved in the Mayo study could move about[57] whereas 17 percent of Dr. Cassileth's patients could not. Yet the Mayo patients had an average median survival of only five months for their cancers compared to sixty-three months for the Cassileth patients. If mobility were a major factor in determining survival outcome, then the Mayo patients should have at least shown survival ratios similar to those in the IAT group.

Problems have also been cited with the age-bias argument. According to Dr. Cassileth, the median age of her patients was "fifty-four years" compared with sixty-one years for conventional cancer patients. This factor is believed to artificially improve the IAT results because younger patients are presumably better able to recover from their cancers. Critics such as Robert Houston, however, charge that Cassileth incorrectly averaged in the lowest possible age of each patient group studied. (For example, in the 40–59-year-old group, age 40 was used as the key number). Houston also points out that the "average" Burton patient seeks therapy seventeen months after diagnosis (and after running the gamut of approved treatments) and is thus older than the median average cited by Dr. Cassileth.

If race and poorer social background enter into the arguments against IAT, then they certainly may be cited as factors in the survival ratios for orthodox cancer treatments as well; national cancer statistics have, in the past, also been based on white survival rates and have excluded blacks, who generally have poorer rates of survival (see Introduction).

Further Criticism of the Cassileth Study

According to Robert Houston, the study's data is presented in such a way as to decrease positive facts but embellish negative ones.

For example, while Dr. Cassileth claims that 33 percent of the IAT patients improved in mobility, Houston found the number actually to be 37 percent.[58] The reason for the discrepancy is that Cassileth averaged into her calculations a number of patients in whom IAT had no effect on mobility. This finding was superfluous, however, because the patients were not considered immobile in the first place.[59]

In another example, 37 percent of Dr. Cassileth's patients were alleged to have died within six months after receiving IAT. But Houston says this number is misleading because 25 patients who died before the study even began were *included* in the final numbers. When this flaw is accounted for, the actual six-month survival becomes 93 percent according to Houston.

Burton's Immuno-Augmentative Therapy is among the most controversial treatments in alternative medicine. Although the ACS disputes this method, some observers cite the preliminary findings of Dr. Cassileth as a vindication of IAT. Nevertheless, there seems to be a general reluctance to give IAT any credit and to blame favorable reports on such factors as "positive biases" and the "placebo affect."

A chief criticism of IAT has been the lack of published data regarding its use, but Burton did publish a study in 1988 showing beneficial results in asbestos-related lung cancer.[60] In this study, Burton reported that IAT-treated patients showed a median survival greater than thirty months—nearly triple the standard survival rate for this type of malignancy.[61] At present, the median survival for patients with asbestos-related lung cancer is only about eleven months.[62]

While national cancer agencies remain skeptical of Dr. Burton's methods, research laboratories in the United States are now developing immune-oriented treatments that are said to be extensions of the very work Burton pioneered. For example, the much publicized drug Interleukin-2 is considered to have conceptual similarities with IAT. In addition, several leading hospitals and universities have been claiming impressive results with "tumor necrosis factor" (TNF)—a protein that causes some cancers to disintegrate in much the same way Burton's serum did in earlier animal experiments.

Perhaps it is no coincidence that TNF, which is made from the same blood protein as Burton's deblocking factor was developed at Sloan-Kettering Cancer Center by one of the original members of Dr. Burton's research team.

For further information contact:

Immuno-Augmentative Therapy
P.O. Box F-2689
Freeport, Grand Bahama Island
(809) 352-7455

IAT Patients' Association
Box 10
Otho, Iowa 50569-0010
(515) 972-4444

SIX

Vitamin C Therapy

In 1966, a Scottish surgeon named Ewan Cameron published a novel theory on how the deadly growth of cancer takes place and how it might be stopped.

Cameron explained that in the human body, a special type of intercellular "cement" made of collagen-like proteins binds the cells and tissues together. Normally, tumors are prevented from growing because of the resilience of these proteins. But Cameron found evidence that malignant tumors release a special enzyme which causes the collagen-like cement to break down. He thus proposed that if a way could be found to reverse this deadly process, a person's natural resistance to cancer would increase. Cameron's efforts then became directed at finding a method to put this theory to the test.

Five years after his thesis was published, Dr. Cameron and the American chemist Linus Pauling theorized that an increased concentration of Vitamin C might inhibit the cement-destroying enzymes as well as strengthen the collagen substance surrounding tumors. Based on this hypothesis, Cameron began treating a small number of seriously ill cancer patients at the Vale of Leven Hospital in Loch Lomonside, Scotland. The dose of vitamin C used in the trial was 10 grams (or 10,000 milligrams). This amount is 165 times the RDA (Recommended Daily Allowance) for an average adult.

Three years after the Vale of Leven trial began, Dr. Cameron reported that patient response was "striking." According to the physician, tumors diminished, patients experienced relief from severe pain and there was less build-up of dangerous fluids associated with tumors. Some "cures" were also being reported.

For the next five years, Cameron and Pauling followed the progress of 100 patients receiving vitamin C at the Vale of Leven. These patients were matched with a 1,000-patient control group receiving only standard therapy. At the conclusion of this trial, Cameron and Pauling reported that the vitamin C patients lived significantly longer than the control group. After announcing their results to the scientific community, a federally sponsored trial on vitamin C was undertaken in 1978 by American physicians at the Mayo Clinic, in Rochester, Minnesota.

The first Mayo study failed to show better survival rates from vitamin C, although improvements in patients' appetites and well-being were noted. But critics quickly found a number of faults with the study, and as a result one more trial was conducted. After this last trial failed to show any benefit, researchers concluded that vitamin C did not improve the survival time of cancer patients.

Based on these negative Mayo results, the American Cancer Society (ACS) considers vitamin C an unproven and ineffective cancer therapy. But Dr. Pauling has remained a severe critic of the Mayo trials and believes the protocols he and Dr. Cameron used in Scotland were never duplicated or followed by the American researchers.

Dr. Cameron's and Dr. Pauling's Credentials

Dr. Ewan Cameron received his medical degree from the University of Glasgow, Scotland. He became a Fellow of the Royal College of Surgeons, Senior Consultant Surgeon at Vale of Leven Hospital, and Civil Consultant in General Surgery to the Royal Navy. He has been honored for achievements in medicine and pathology.[1]

Dr. Linus Pauling received his Ph.D. in Chemistry from the California Institute of Technology (Caltech) in 1925. He was then granted a National Research Fellowship and a Guggenheim Fellowship. While furthering his studies at the Institute for Theoretical

Physics in Munich, Pauling began exploring novel concepts in quantum physics, then in its infancy. After returning from Europe, Pauling became a lecturer and research chemist at Caltech.

In 1939, Dr. Pauling wrote *The Nature of the Chemical Bond and the Structure of Molecules and Crystals.* This work has been considered one of the most "influential" science texts "ever written."[2] More than a decade later, Pauling became one of the first scientists to conceptualize how DNA—the master molecule of life—was constructed.[3] His theories were said to have preceded Francis H. C. Crick's and James D. Watson's discovery of DNA by one year. For his research efforts, Pauling was awarded the Nobel Prize for Chemistry in 1954.

In 1962, the scientist became an outspoken critic of nuclear testing and for this effort, was again awarded the Nobel Prize, this time for peace. In 1967, the controversial scientist accepted an appointment as research professor of chemistry at the University of California in San Diego and became actively involved in the role of vitamins and other micronutrients on health. Soon after, his first general health book *Vitamin C and the Common Cold*, won the Phi Beta Kappa Award for the most important work of general science that year.

According to an article appearing in the acclaimed journal *Scientific American*, Pauling is considered a "supreme theorist and experimentalist" who helped "lay the foundation of modern chemistry, biochemistry and molecular biology."[4] Even greater accolades were paid by the British journal *New Scientist*, which calls Pauling one of the twenty greatest scientists "of all time"—on a par with Newton, Darwin, and Einstein.[5]

In his nineties, the Nobel laureate is currently president of the Linus Pauling Institute of Science and Medicine in Menlo Park, California.

Supporting Vitamin C's Use in Cancer Treatment

Pauling and Cameron were influenced by a number of medical reports that suggested a therapeutic role for ascorbic acid (i.e., vitamin C) in cancer treatment.

As early as 1753, an anatomist described a close parallel between scurvy—a disease caused by vitamin C deficiency—and the frequency of malignant tumors.[6] Pauling felt that although the scurvy report was outdated, it might have significance.

After further investigation, Pauling discovered a 1937 study which further established a link between blood levels of vitamin C and cancer susceptibility. In the study, it was noted that healthy people had normal vitamin ranges in their blood but for cancer patients, the levels were abnormally low.[7] In their own experiments, Pauling and Cameron also found that cancer patients had unusually low amounts of ascorbic acid in their disease-fighting white blood cells.[8] Interestingly, these levels dropped even lower if patients were receiving surgery or radiation for their cancer.

Pauling concluded that toxic cancer therapies actually cause people to lose more vitamin C than they take in and this results in a "fairly severe ascorbic acid deficiency."[9] He and Cameron reasoned that a vitamin C imbalance

> interferes with the healing processes and with the body's immune resistance not only to cancer but against any intercurrent infection, and contributes to complications and the overall debility of the 'cancer-plus-treatment' illness.[10]

Based on all these considerations, Cameron and Pauling were convinced that vitamin C would prove useful in the treatment of cancer. They decided to launch a clinical trial involving human cancer patients in 1973.

The Vale of Leven Trials

Originally, a randomized, double-blind trial was planned; in this type of study, one group of patients receives the actual treatment and the other group, a placebo or "dummy" pill having no medical value. But Dr. Cameron had become so convinced of the curative value of vitamin C that he could not agree to a random study on moral grounds.[11] In view of this objection, Cameron and Pauling decided on conducting a *retrospective trial* in which they would match and compare every one of their vitamin C-treated cancer patients with ten other patients receiving only standard therapy in the same hospital. The hospital patients, though not active participants in the vitamin C study, would serve as "controls."[12]

According to the Vale of Leven researchers, their control group was

obtained by a random search of the case record index of similar patients treated by the same clinicians in the Vale of Leven Hospital...For each [vitamin C] treated patient, 10 controls were found of the same sex, within 5 years of the same age, and who had suffered from cancer of the same primary organ and...tumor type.[13]

To insure accuracy, Pauling and Cameron employed an independent physician with no previous knowledge of the study patients to assess the treatment results.

The Vale of Leven Trial Results

In 1976, Cameron and Pauling published the long-awaited results of their Vale of Leven trial. In an article which appeared in the medical journal *Proceedings of the National Academy of Sciences*,[14] the researchers announced that 1,000 control patients who received standard therapies had died by completion of the three-year trial. But the vitamin C patients lived an average of 300 days *longer* than their counterparts. Further, 18 of the vitamin C-group patients survived four times longer than would be commonly expected—beyond what Pauling describes as the point of "untreatability" (see Figure 1).

Pauling and Cameron also compared their vitamin-treated patients with controls according to type of cancer. The researchers claimed that

Figure 1
Vale of Leven Study Results

Survival Time From Start of Study (days)	Vitamin C group (% still alive)	Controls
50	67%	36%
100	53	12
200	28	2.5
300	18	1.7
400	16	0.3
500	11	—
600	7	—

there were highly measurable differences among survival rates for such untreatable cancers as those of the stomach and lung (see Figure 2).

Figure 2
Survival Time for Specific Types of Cancers
After Time of Untreatability

Number of Days After Point of Untreatability	Cancer Type	Survival % for vitamin C group	Survival % controls
100	Colon	80%	9%
500		35	0
100	Stomach	52	8
500		8	0
100	Lung	50	5
500		5	0
100	Breast	65	20
500		42	1

Other Independent Trials of Vitamin C and Cancer

In 1979, Japanese scientists conducted a vitamin C-cancer study at the Fukuoka Torikai Hospital in Fukuoka, Japan. Unlike the Scottish trial, the Japanese patients did not all uniformly receive 10 grams of vitamin C. Instead, some received 4 grams or less, and others 5 grams or more, averaging as high as 29 grams daily. In a report which appeared in the *Journal of the International Academy of Preventive Medicine*, the researchers noted that patients receiving the lowest vitamin amounts did not survive longer than 174 days, whereas 33 percent of the high-dose group lived beyond that time frame.[15]

In the laboratory, scientists also showed that vitamin C could selectively kill certain types of deadly cancer cells in the test tube.[16]

The National Cancer Institute and the Vitamin C Investigation

In 1973, Dr. Pauling met with scientists at the National Cancer Institute (NCI) in Bethesda, Maryland, to discuss the possibility of launching a prospective trial on vitamin C. NCI officials did not agree to one, and it was not until five years later that Dr. Vincent DeVita, a former director of the institute, authorized a vitamin trial.

In 1978, the first American trial on vitamin C was conducted at the Mayo Clinic under the supervision of Dr. Charles Moertel. (Moertel was also the primary investigator in the unsuccessful Laetrile studies at the Mayo Clinic).

One hundred twenty-three patients who all had "biopsy-proven advanced and incurable cancers" of either the abdomen or lung were selected for the study.[17] Sixty patients received 10 grams of vitamin C daily and 63, a placebo tablet with no medical value. The patients were all carefully matched for age, weight, sex, and types of cancers. While some of the patients were disabled, only a small amount were considered "bedridden."[18]

According to a report which later appeared in the *New England Journal of Medicine*,[19] no appreciable difference was noted in survival time between both groups of patients, and, ironically, the longest-surviving patient was one who had received only the placebo.[20] For a while, these results were believed to put the vitamin C controversy to rest.

In a statement delivered shortly after the Mayo results were announced, Dr. Pauling argued that the trial did not accurately duplicate his and Cameron's own study. Pauling complained that the patients had almost all received prior courses of chemotherapy before receiving vitamin C. Because Pauling and Cameron were convinced that chemotherapy traumatizes the immune system,[21] they felt that the Mayo patients were already compromised beyond the point of treatability.

Doctors disagreed, saying that advanced cancer patients who had received toxic drug therapies in previous studies were shown to have functioning immune systems.[22] Further, they claimed that the Vale of Leven patients had also received standard therapies.[23] In reply, Pauling stated that toxic drug therapy was only "rarely" used to treat patients in Scotland and of his 100 patients, only 4 had received any course of previous therapy.[24]

In response to Pauling's objections, the NCI decided to retest vitamin C.

In the second study, 100 patients with "tissue proven" cancer of the colon were admitted to the Mayo Clinic for a second trial. The patients were "beyond any hope of a curative therapy" but could move about without help.[25] Fifty-one of the patients were randomly selected to receive vitamin C and the remaining 49, a placebo. As one condition of the study, vitamin C would be discontinued as soon as any deterioration or decrease in patient health was noted.[26]

To address Dr. Pauling's earlier objections, the Mayo team selected volunteers who had not had any previous chemotherapy.[27] Also, to be sure that the placebo patients were not taking vitamin C on their own, Moertel and colleagues took routine urine samples.

After several months of observation, the Mayo researchers announced their findings. They concluded that, overall:

—Those patients having measurable tumors showed no objective regression regardless of the group they were in.

—The same number of people experienced relief from symptoms, regardless of the group they were in.

—Among those patients whose cancers progressed after starting the study, no differences were found between the placebo and control groups.

—The "median survival" for all patients was about $10^1/_2$ months.

Dr. Pauling and Others Again Challenge the Mayo Clinic's Findings

Because the Mayo Clinic patients were only given vitamin C for two months and not indefinitely (as in the Vale of Leven study), Dr. Pauling objected that there was not enough time to assess possible benefits. Further, vitamin C was abruptly withdrawn at the first sign of a downturn in health; if anything, argued Pauling, the vitamin should have been administered in even larger doses.

Another major objection to the Mayo trials was the possibility of test "cheating." As already mentioned, urine samples were checked to determine whether patients in the placebo group were self-medicating. The Moertel researchers were satisfied that they were not. Independent critics, however, have charged that the Moertel report raises troubling questions over its own conclusions.

For example, some of the control patients were found to be excreting about 500 milligrams (equaling one half-gram) or more of vitamin C daily.[28] It is generally recognized that by eating a balanced diet, an average adult would, under normal circumstances, eliminate only about 10 milligrams—or 2 percent of the amount being passed by the control patients. To excrete 500 milligrams, an individual would have to take in about 2 grams of vitamin C daily—a fairly large amount that is usually gotten only by deliberate supplementation.[29]

Pauling warned Mayo scientists that abrupt cessation of vitamin C could actually result in a dangerously low level of the substance, leading to a deterioration in the patients.[30] This warning was based on a phenomenon known as the "rebound effect."

According to Pauling, special enzymes are used by the body to help utilize vitamin C. The greater the amount of vitamin a person takes in, the more enzymes are needed to break it down. Consequently, when large doses of vitamin C are suddenly discontinued, an increased load of enzymes overcompensates and vitamin levels then drop below normal. This effect is believed to actually cause a *worsening* of the disease being treated.

Pauling argued that this scenario may have occurred when the Mayo doctors suddenly discontinued treatment as soon as patients showed signs of worsening.

Again, Pauling pushed for a third, lengthier trial in which he and Dr. Moertel would collaborate and reach an agreement on specifics, Moertel, however, refused to retest vitamin C.

The Mayo Clinic Researchers are Accused of "Fraud"

Pauling claims that Dr. Moertel, a spokesman for the National Cancer Institute (NCI) and the editor of the *New England Journal of Medicine* (*NEJM*) deliberately prevented him and Cameron from "obtaining any information" about the Mayo results until just "a few hours before publication."[31] In Pauling's view, this was an attempt to discourage him from pointing out flaws in the trial before it became public. Pauling also claims that Dr. Moertel promised to share the trial results with him six weeks before the *NEJM* report was made public but then reneged on his promise. According to Pauling, these breaches of professional ethics prevented a fair and objective report on vitamin C, and the subsequent report was thus fraudulent.

While Pauling's accusations may appear extreme, there *is* evidence that he was prevented from publishing a rebuttal to the Moertel article.[32] And when the Nobel laureate protested, he was apparently ignored. In a letter to the editor of *NEJM*, Pauling wrote:

> some time ago I wrote to you, asking for information about the process by which this fraudulent paper came to be accepted for publication in your journal. You have not answered my letter. I hope that you will do one the courtesy of answering my letter. Your continued failure to do so would indicate that you also are involved in this conspiracy to suppress the truth.[33]

In 1989, Dr. Pauling finally did manage to have his rebuttal published and it appeared in the *Proceedings of the National Academy of Sciences*.[34]

Other Studies on Vitamin C and Malignant Diseases

During the late 1980s, Dr. Pauling petitioned the NCI to consider a third trial of vitamin C. But the request was denied because of concern that any possible long-term effects of vitamin C would not show up in a standard trial.[35] Pauling did convince NCI officials to sponsor a conference on vitamin C research, which was held in 1990 at the National Institutes of Health (NIH).[36] A number of distinguished researchers from around the world attended and presented dozens of scientific papers.

In general, orthodox scientists appeared reticent to speculate on vitamin C's therapeutic role in cancer, but they admitted that the "status" of this controversial substance "has changed in a lot of researchers' minds."[37] For the most part, the 1990 conference centered on vitamin C's crucial role in cancer prevention as well as in other terminal diseases, including AIDS.

Although the majority of vitamin C reports discussed at the NIH dealt with areas other than cancer treatment, a few favorable studies emerged. For example, vitamin C was shown to inhibit malignant cell division in mice[38] and possibly to serve as a useful adjunct in the treatment of advanced cancer in people.[39]

In other areas of study, researchers expressed surprise at the vitamin's potential usefulness in helping cancer patients cope with the disastrous effects of conventional chemotherapy.[40] For instance, Japanese researchers found that vitamin C can offer protective affects against Adriamycin—a commonly used cancer drug known to damage heart muscle and even result in fatal cardiac arrest.[41] In addition, investigators from Montefiore Medical Center in New York discovered that patients undergoing treatment with the experimental cancer drug Interleukin-2 could benefit from vitamin C supplementation because these patients experience a drastic ascorbate deficiency akin to scurvy.[42] This finding coincides with some of Pauling's earlier claims.

Ironically, while vitamin C remains highly controversial as a form of therapy for cancer (and most other diseases as well), its theoretical role in cancer prevention has become almost universally accepted. According to the NCI's chief of the Cancer Prevention Division, "when you eat foods that are high in vitamin C, you have a lower risk of cancer"[43]; this fact is apparently "well established" even among traditional scientists.[44]

One reason that vitamin C may be able to prevent cancer lies in its unique ability to neutralize free radicals.* In fact, vitamin C has been shown to be one of the most powerful "antioxidants" available.[45]

Research on Vitamin C and AIDS

Besides its effects against cancer, ascorbic acid has also been shown to inhibit the devastating AIDS virus in the test tube.[46] One physician has reported dramatic improvements in AIDS patients and the diseases plaguing them after intravenous administration of vitamin C in doses as high as 60 to 180 grams.[47]

The only positive cancer studies on vitamin C to date have been performed at the Vale of Leven hospital and the Fukuoka Torikai Hospital in Japan. While the Mayo Clinic trials were negative, it is possible that variances in study duration account for the contradictory results. A careful inspection of the survival graphs in Figure 3 illustrates this point.

Viewed as a whole, the vitamin C-treated patients show a more favorable curve than the controls. At many places, however, both curves dip in the same direction. Depending on the point in time one chooses to view the curves, they might appear either similar (i.e., heading in the same direction), or distinctly different. Since the Mayo

---

*Electrically charged molecules which can form when fats are oxidized in the body. Free radicals have been linked to aging, heart disease, and cancer.

trials were of far shorter duration than the Vale of Leven study, no one can say what the Mayo results would have been had the tracking curves been allowed to continue indefinitely.

Figure 3
Survival Graph for Incurable Cancer Patients Receiving Vitamin C vs. Untreated Controls

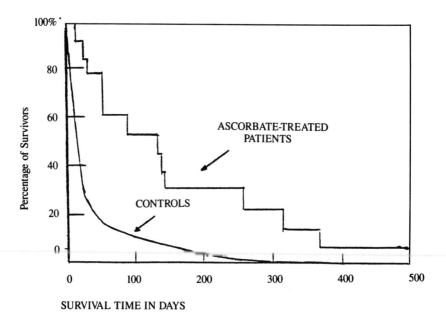

SURVIVAL TIME IN DAYS

Source: Linus Pauling Institute of Science and Medicine

In the absence of any incontrovertible data which refutes Dr. Pauling's findings, one of two possible conclusions can be drawn: Either his study was accurate and the vitamin C-treated cancer patients benefited remarkably, or the study was terribly flawed and all the positive results were merely statistical blunders.

While the first conclusion remains speculative, many observers dispute the "statistical blunder" argument on the grounds that Dr. Pauling's internationally acclaimed reputation as a Nobel laureate lends at least *some* degree of validity to his claims.

Despite the controversy, vitamin C's relative safety, accessibility, and inexpense make it readily available for those considering using it. Most proponents, however, would probably agree that the vitamin should not be considered a sole treatment modality but as a useful adjunct to other standard or alternative therapies.

For those interested in a high-dose vitamin C program, several precautions should be taken into account.

Vitamin C exists in different forms—the most common being ascorbic acid. However, the salt version (known as *sodium ascorbate*) may cause problems. For example, people on salt-restricted diets can experience adverse effects. In addition, one study has shown that high-dose administration of sodium ascorbate actually *promoted* cancer growth in experimental animals.[48] But in another study, it was found that it is only the salt and *not* the ascorbic acid version that may cause problems.

In other cases, high-dose vitamin C may interact with and affect such medications as Coumadin—a blood-thinning drug.[49] Therefore, anyone considering vitamin C therapy should consult with a nutritionally oriented or orthomolecular** physician experienced in its use.

For further information contact:

Linus Pauling Institute of Science and Medicine
440 Page Mill Road
Palo Alto, CA 94306
(415) 327-4064

Center for Metabolic Disorders
5030 90th Way S.W.
Fort Lauderdale, FL 33328
(305) 929-4814

Michael B. Schachter, M.D.
Two Executive Blvd.
Suite 202
Suffern, NY 10901
(914) 368-4700

**Orthomolecular physicians treat and prevent diseases by administering the correct levels of micronutrients. Based on individual requirements, the doses given can exceed hundreds of times the recommended daily allowances.

SEVEN

Laetrile

Laetrile is the synthetic version of a natural substance known as *amygdalin*; amygdalin is found in plants, seeds, and nuts and under certain conditions, can yield cyanide.

Amygdalin was first purified from bitter almonds in 1830 by two French scientists. One cancer patient was then given an extract of the substance and reported cured.[1] More than a century later, Dr. Ernest Krebs, Jr., of San Francisco developed a method to synthesize Laetrile and then proposed a controversial theory on how it might arrest tumor growth.

Krebs hypothesized that cancer tissues have high concentrations of a substance known as *beta-glucosidase*; he maintained that through a series of chemical interactions, beta-glucosidase causes the release of cyanide from Laetrile, and malignant cells are then destroyed. Fortunately, healthy cells contain a substance known as *rhodanese* and it, said Krebs, "neutralizes" the effects of cyanide. If this theory were true, then Laetrile would represent the first drug which could selectively target malignant cells but spare healthy ones; in effect, Laetrile would be the "magic bullet" scientists have long been searching for.

To test his hypothesis, Krebs combined beta-glucosidase with Laetrile in a test tube and reported smelling the familiar almond scent of cyanide. Then, he injected himself with Laetrile and experienced no ill effects. Krebs conducted further experiments and claimed that he could shrink animal tumors with the substance. Later, a number of human cancer cures were reported.

The American Cancer Society (ACS) disagrees with Krebs and discounts the rationale for using Laetrile in human cancer.

In fact, many scientists agree that Dr. Krebs made crucial errors in his theories on how Laetrile is supposed to work. For example, independent research suggests that cancer cells do not contain any more beta-glucosidase than normal tissues and are thus not more vulnerable to the release of cyanide.[2] In addition, a federally sponsored scientific trial of Laetrile was said to show no appreciable improvement in people with cancer. For these reasons, the ACS calls Krebs's theories and the entire premise of Laetrile therapy a "fallacy."[3] As a result, Laetrile is considered a worthless drug and is on the ACS *Unproven Therapies List.*

Scientific Proof in Support of Laetrile

Conflicting reports in the literature lend some support to Krebs's theories. For example, while the ACS is adamant that cancer cells do not contain more beta-glucosidase than normal tissues, Sloan-Kettering scientists did find higher levels of this enzyme.[4]

Other scientists feel that while Krebs's theories do contain errors, cyanide release does occur from Laetrile and this can influence the destruction of cancer cells.

According to Dr. Mark McCarty of the University of California School of Medicine, Laetrile when taken orally, is converted into cyanide in the intestines. Cyanide levels then increase in the body and may have a range of anticancer effects. These effects include the disruption of sugars used by tumors and the activation of "suicide bags" found in malignant cells.[5]

In addition to the mechanism of cyanide, Laetrile contains a number of other substances that may inhibit cancer.

Two studies conducted in 1977 and 1981 have shown, for example, that cancer growth can be blocked by a number of naturally occurring plant substances which are chemically related to Laetrile.[6] Laetrile-like compounds have also been shown to have *antioxidant* properties;

many researchers think that antioxidants (which "scavenge" or dispose of unhealthy molecules in the body) play useful roles in cancer treatment and prevention.[7]

Early Trials of Laetrile

In the 1950s, several physicians claimed that patients benefited from Laetrile therapy.

One of the first doctors to test the drug was Dr. Arthur Harris, a native of South Africa. Harris's first patient was a thirty-six-year-old woman suffering from cervical cancer which had been confirmed via biopsy. Surgery or other known therapies were rejected due to the woman's condition. Several months after starting Laetrile therapy, a second set of biopsies and tests showed "no evidence" of cancer. By all accounts, the woman's previously "eroding cervix" had completely healed.[8]

During the next few years, Harris treated an additional 82 patients. Of these, 24 were said to have remained in remission after ten years and 3 were reportedly cured.[9]

An Italian researcher from the University of Turin claimed yet further evidence in favor of Laetrile. After treating patients with cancers of the uterus, cervix, rectum, and breast, Dr. Ettore Guidetti concluded that the "effects produced by Laetrile on [cancers] appear to confirm [the] chemotherapeutic action" of the drug.[10] He also noted that when Laetrile was applied directly to cancerous tissues, there was an absolute "destructive effect" to the tumor, with a regression of cancer.[11]

National cancer agencies reviewed these early Laetrile reports. But medical experts disputed them because people allegedly being cured by Laetrile were not part of carefully controlled studies which pair treated with nontreated patients.

In addition, a special committee named the California Cancer Commission (CCC) launched an investigation into Laetrile in April of 1953 and concluded that the drug was completely ineffective against cancer.[12] Because the CCC was considered a highly distinguished medical committee, its conclusions would have a long-ranging impact on the Laetrile issue for decades to come. Even as late as 1988, the ACS referred to the CCC reports in drawing its own negative conclusions about Laetrile.

The two primary authors of the CCC report were doctors Ian MacDonald and Henry Garland.

Initially, both MacDonald and Garland categorically stated that examinations of Laetrile-treated patients showed that tumors were not being destroyed by the drug. But in a memorandum made public ten years later, one pathologist who had testified to the CCC during the drafting of its report stated that he had observed such effects as hemorrhaging, necrosis (i.e., dying) and a degeneration of tumor cells after Laetrile treatment. The pathologist attributed these effects to the possible chemical properties of Laetrile.[13]

There is also evidence that MacDonald and Garland may have ignored other key facts in their assessment of Laetrile. For example, in a statement issued on Jan. 14, 1953, researchers confirmed Krebs's original finding that Laetrile can release cyanide under specific conditions. But Garland and MacDonald apparently ignored this report and quoted, instead, the statement of a Dr. John W. Mehl who said that cyanide cannot be released from Laetrile.*[14] Since the issue over cyanide release was crucial to the entire value of Laetrile therapy, Mehl's conclusion had dealt a serious blow to proponents of the drug.

According to Laetrile activist and author Ed Griffin, MacDonald and Garland had gone on record passing questionable judgments on other aspects of medical research only to be proved wrong later on. For example, in a speech given in San Francisco, Garland argued that cigarettes were not a major cause of lung cancer and even joked that cigarettes are "one of the better tranquilizers."[15] At the time of Garland's speech, a strong suspicion between smoking and cancer had already been established and had become a major source of interest to researchers.[16]

Dr. MacDonald was himself quoted in *U.S. News & World Report* in 1957 as stating that "a pack a day keeps lung cancer away."[17] Later, the most remarkable of ironies befell the CCC authors: Dr. MacDonald died in a fire started by his own lighted cigarette, and Dr. Garland died of lung cancer.[18]

Yet even after the CCC report was issued, a number of physicians continued claiming highly favorable benefits from Laetrile. In 1957, Dr. Manuel Navarro, a professor of Medicine and Surgery at the

---

*It is now common knowledge that Laetrile can release cyanide. Several cyanide-related deaths have, in fact, been reported and are cited as reasons *against* using the drug.

University of Santo Tomas in Manila, announced that when he administered Laetrile to fourteen advanced cancer patients, there was a "striking relief of pain with the discontinuance of analgesics [pain killers], disappearance of fetor [odor] from ulcerations, improved appetite and regression of tumor."[19] After treating over 500 patients, Navarro concluded that Laetrile caused "encouraging and significant results."[20]

In a European study involving twenty-one people dying from cancer, treatment with Laetrile was said to effect the relief of pain and a reduction of hemorrhage and jaundice, significant and constant improvement in strength, and in some cases an appreciable reduction of malignant tumors.[21]

In 1962, Dr. John Morrone, an attending surgeon at the Jersey City Medical Center, treated ten terminally ill cancer patients with Laetrile; all the patients had been described as having "inoperable" cancer. While no cures were effected, Morrone claimed results similar to Navarro and his European colleagues.[22] According to Morrone, intravenous injections of Laetrile resulted in a "dramatic relief of pain." In most cases, narcotics were discontinued and swelling was considerably reduced.[23]

Dr. Morrone concluded: "It would appear that Laetrile...causes a regression of the malignant lesion."[24]

Sloan-Kettering Cancer Center's Investigation of Laetrile

Most of Sloan-Kettering's research on Laetrile was performed by Dr. Kanematsu Sugiura, a senior professor emeritus and one of the center's most experienced research authorities. Sugiura had also authored hundreds of scientific articles on cancer.

During Sugiura's first few months of studying Laetrile, he found that the drug significantly inhibited the appearance of lung tumors in mice. In addition, the researcher found that Laetrile prevented the development of spontaneous cancers which normally occur in some experimental animals.[25] Sugiura also noted that other cancer drugs had never caused complete regressions in the tumors being studied, as Laetrile had.[26]

In view of these impressive reports, Sloan-Kettering officials began organizing a task force to assess the drug. Plans were also drawn to bring other members of the alternative-cancer community together as part of the task force. But one year after the plan was drafted, support for Laetrile within the cancer center collapsed.

Fearing that Sloan-Kettering was about to "close the books" on Laetrile, concerned employees formed a watchdog group they named "Second Opinion." The group's key organizer was Ralph Moss, then director of communications at the center.

Second Opinion tried to persuade officials to reconsider testing Laetrile. But when that failed, the upstart group issued an unauthorized bulletin to the press in the form of scientific data, test results, and notes compiled by Dr. Sugiura. As a result of this press leak, Ralph Moss was fired.[27] But Sloan-Kettering *did* yield to another investigation and this time sponsored a trial which included Sugiura and another researcher, Dr. Franz Schmid. Once again, Laetrile was said to have effected a favorable outcome against cancer in animals, and this prompted a San Francisco reporter to call the latest results "dramatic...."[28] But according to Moss, Schmid refused to comment on the tests and appeared unwilling to verify the results.

Sloan-Kettering officials argued that Dr. Sugiura had conducted faulty studies because he did not use "control animals" as a means of comparing his Laetrile results; he was also said to have "mistakenly" formed his judgment on the drug's effects by measuring tumor shrinkage "visually."[29] Further, another series of animal tests, which were performed by Dr. Daniel S. Martin of the Catholic Medical Center in Queens, reportedly showed that Laetrile did not shrink tumors.

Sugiura complained that Dr. Martin's negative results were flawed because only one cage was used to house both the untreated controls and the animals being given Laetrile. Sugiura argued that this was poor scientific practice because the control animals could easily have been mistaken for the Laetrile-treated ones. In fact, some the controls even experienced *more* tumor regression than their treated counterparts, further raising Sugiura's suspicions.[30] Despite these inconsistencies and the number of earlier studies performed by Sugiura, Sloan-Kettering announced that Laetrile testing had failed on all counts.

Based on the negative Sloan-Kettering studies and other reports, the ACS concluded that Laetrile was without benefit against animal tumors.

Independent Laetrile Studies

Several independent laboratories in the United States and abroad claimed to have found evidence that Laetrile caused definite antitumor activity in animals.

In a series of experiments conducted at the Southern Research Institute in Birmingham, Alabama, a majority of 280 mice with lung cancer were said to have responded favorably to Laetrile.[31] In another series of studies performed at the SCIND Laboratories at the University of San Francisco, 80 percent of 400 rats with cancer experienced a significant increase in lifespan after receiving Laetrile; this study prompted the director of the National Cancer Institute (NCI) to write: "The data certainly indicates some activity in animal tumor systems."[32]

At the Pasteur Institute in Paris, 100 percent animal remissions were announced with Laetrile. And in Germany, a significant delay of cancer incidence and increased life span in mice was also reported[33].

In 1976, two veterinarians had also published articles in peer-review journals documenting remission of cancer in dogs and cats as a result of Laetrile therapy.[34]

The Effect of Laetrile on Humans

In the wake of considerable public pressure, the NCI agreed to conduct clinical trials of Laetrile in 1979. The study enlisted 178 people with advanced cancer for "whom no other means of therapy" could offer any "further benefit."[35] The patients were all able to eat and could walk about with help. Seventy percent were still able to work.[36]

The NCI said that the Laetrile it used was "prepared from apricot pits and corresponded to the products distributed by the major Mexican supplier of Laetrile, American Biologics. The drug's purity was established by extensive assays."[37]

In addition to recommended doses of Laetrile, the trial patients all received an "overall metabolic therapy program consisting of vitamins... [and] minerals..." as prescribed by current Laetrile practitioners.[38] Diet was restricted, and the use of "eggs, meat, refined-flour products, caffeine and alcohol were prohibited. Fresh fruits, vegetables and whole grains were emphasized."[39]

Three months after the trials began, the NCI made the following observation: cancer "had progressed in 90 percent of patients. By eight months, 80 percent were dead. These results are similar to those found with no treatment." The study authors concluded that:

> no substantive benefit was observed in terms of cure, improvement or stabilization of cancer, improvement of symptoms related to cancer, or extension of life span.

The ACS thus concluded that the 1979 trial showed "unequivocally that Laetrile is ineffective for cancer therapy." But Laetrile supporters immediately voiced their protest over the way the NCI trials were conducted. The primary criticisms included the following:

1. All of the people chosen for the NCI trials were listed as "phase IV"—i.e., patients with incurable cancer for whom no hope of a cure existed. Critics thus charged that the NCI study was biased because Laetrile could hardly have helped people already given up as beyond the hope of any therapy, conventional or otherwise, to cure them.

2. The Laetrile used in the study was not "real" Laetrile. According to Greg Kaye, founder of the New Jersey Freedom of Choice Committee and president of Cyto Metabolics Inc. in Linden, New Jersey, the "NCI failed to meet" (the) specifications for establishing the purity and potency of the drug that it tested. Kaye stated that the NCI was "well aware of the clinical differences and lack of efficacy of this substance, as a confidential memo in my [Kaye's] possession from Dr. Moertel [the NCI trial director] on Mayo Clinic stationery [dated Feb. 14, 1979] will document."[40]

3. Some patients did, in fact, improve in the study, but these were not quoted in the popular media, according to Michael Culbert, president of The Committee for Freedom of Choice in Medicine, Inc., and noted historian on the Laetrile controversy. Culbert states that two sets of trial data were actually disseminated—one to the public *before* the NCI trial was over and a final evaluation which escaped media attention. Culbert says that according to a *New England Journal of Medicine* report, either a "small majority or a large minority of these... terminal patients were

either 'stable' or had 'no measurable progression of malignant disease' as long as they continued receiving intravenous Laetrile.[41] Culbert also adds that after twenty-one days, the intravenous Laetrile was stopped and patients were then continued on oral amygdalin.[42]

Laetrile's Toxicity

It is well established that overdoses of Laetrile can cause cyanide toxicity and even death—especially when the drug is taken orally.

The ACS cites an example of a person who developed muscular weakness and respiratory problems from taking Laetrile. Another patient who was not under a doctor's care died from apparent cyanide poisoning after Laetrile ingestion. Other cases of adverse reactions have also been documented.

Michael Culbert dismisses these reports as pure "propaganda artifice," explaining that Laetrile's safety has already been proved by virtue of its not causing any problems in the 1979 NCI trial. Former communications director Ralph Moss adds that tens upon thousands of people have used and continue using the drug worldwide and, of these, cyanide toxicity has only occurred in a miniscule amount and generally in those not being monitored by qualified physicians. Other critics argue that no cancer drug is without side effects, and they cite the established number of fatalities that occur yearly from their use.

The only federally approved clinical trial of Laetrile to date concluded with negative results and is considered a prima facie case against the drug. Laetrile supporters argue, however, that the NCI trial patients were deemed beyond the hope of *any* therapy to cure them—standard or otherwise; since Laetrile is now believed to work best against earlier stage cancers and in combination with other alternative therapies, proponents argue that further studies will be necessary to assess the drug conclusively. But given the official position against Laetrile, it is a virtual certainty that such studies will never take place.

When asked why the Laetrile trial did not include a control group, NCI researchers replied that it would be "unconscionable to randomize people between a [worthless] drug [i.e., Laetrile]...and standard therapy that [might extend life]." Critics, however, see this statement as an admission of study bias, for if another therapy that could extend life was in fact available, why was it withheld from the NCI trial patients? The obvious answer, say the critics, is that no such therapy existed which could help the incurable patients.

Theoretically, Laetrile could still be tested and evaluated by using the benefit of a control group. One way to avoid any legal or ethical problems would be to give the drug adjunctively to a group of cancer patients treated with the usual standard therapies. Then, via computer matching, a similar group of patients receiving only standard treatments would be used as the controls.

Whatever the outcome of such a study, it is generally accepted by most observers that Laetrile—by itself—is not a cancer cure. For specific, treatable cancers, however, it remains to be seen whether the drug may or may not extend life span when used as part of a broader program of therapy. In this regard, a number of "metabolic" clinics (as listed throughout this book) routinely use Laetrile in combination with any number of modalities. The majority of American physicians as well as the American Cancer Society would be decidedly against the notion that such a program might incur possible benefits. But while the ACS states that "no evidence" has ever shown Laetrile to be effective, numerous examples—including the Scind experiments and Sugiura studies—appear to show otherwise.

Interestingly, in a questionnaire sent to nearly a half-million physicians, the ACS admits that "*only* [emphasis mine] 93 'positive' outcomes" from Laetrile therapy were reported. The ACS does not explain how many physicians responded to the inquiry nor does it explain *why* the 93 cancer patients received benefit from a drug it says is completely worthless.

For further information contact:

American Biologics**
1180 Walnut Avenue
Chula Vista, CA 91911
(619) 429-8200
(800) 227-4473

**Most metabolic cancer clinics offer Laetrile as an integral part of their overall treatment program.

Vladimir Rizov, M.D.
8311 Shoal Creek Blvd.
Austin, TX 78758
(512) 451-8149

Gibson Clinic of Preventive Medicine
215 North Third Street
Ponca City, OK 74601
(405) 762-5746

EIGHT

Burzynski's Antineoplastons

In the 1970s, a Polish biochemist named Stanislaw Burzynski attracted worldwide attention when he claimed that clusters of amino acids known as "peptides" could block the growth of cancer cells.

After immigrating to the United States and taking on a prestigious position at Baylor College of Medicine in Houston, Texas, Burzynski developed his theories and then named his peptides "*antineoplastons.*" Some studies involving animals suggested that antineoplastons could stop the growth of tumors. And trials involving people were also said to have been impressive. In 1977, Dr. Burzynski left Baylor, established a clinic known as the Burzynski Research Institute (BRI), and then began treating cancer patients.

Since the BRI has been in operation, there has been heated debate over the validity of antineoplastons to treat cancer. Critics argue that antineoplastons have not shown any effect against animal and human cancers. Further, Dr. Burzynski has been blamed for promoting unscientific theories and for breaching ethical propriety by administering an unapproved and expensive drug to humans. As a result, a series of lawsuits have been taken against BRI by the state of Texas.

In response to what they consider a vicious propaganda campaign, hundreds of cancer patients have come forward and launched a crusade to help "Dr. B" as they affectionately call Burzynski. Hundreds of supportive letters were mailed to the governor of Texas and other legislators. This effort was further backed by a nonprofit advocacy group known as the "Patient Legal Action Fund," which has joined in the legal battle to defend and represent Dr. Burzynski.

At this time, the American Cancer Society (ACS) does not consider antineoplastons effective against cancer and urges that patients not use this therapy. However, in the wake of recent scientific findings which have validated Burzynski's work, both the National Cancer Institute (NCI) and the Food and Drug Administration (FDA) have granted permission to launch clinical trials of antineoplastons. This unexpected turnaround has resulted, in part, from a favorable review of patients with advanced brain cancer treated with the controversial drug.

Dr. Burzynski's Credentials

Dr. Stanislaw R. Burzynski was born in Poland in 1943 and received all of his formal education in that country. In 1968 he earned his medical degree from the Academy of Lublin. After completing his residency in internal medicine, the physician continued studies in advanced biochemistry and later received a doctoral degree in that subject.

In 1970, Burzynski immigrated to the United States and settled in Texas. There, he was accepted as a research associate in the Department of Anesthesiology at Baylor College of Medicine in Houston.[1] Three years after selection to this post, the physician became licensed to practice medicine in the United States by the Texas board of Medical Examiners. Burzynski was then named assistant professor of medicine at Baylor and remained there until 1977. Later, the Polish emigré became head of the Burzynski Research Institute in Houston.[2]

How Dr. Burzynski Developed his Cancer Treatment

Early in his research, Dr. Burzynski studied the role that peptides might play in memory retention. After conducting several experiments,[3, 4] he formulated an intriguing theory on the possible connection between peptides and cancer.

Burzynski postulated that peptide molecules could carry or store information.[5] This information serves a number of different purposes, including regulation of cell growth. Because Burzynski claimed to find evidence that cancer patients lack certain peptides in their blood, he concluded that the missing molecules play a crucial role in both the causation and possible cure of cancer.

Based on this concept, Burzynski felt that an ideal approach in treating cancer would be to "redirect" malignant cells into normal behavior patterns by giving people the correct amounts of missing peptides or, as he later named them, antineoplastons.

During this time, Burzynski also advanced the idea of a "Biochemical Defense System" (BDI). According to his theory, the BDI is similar to the immune system but instead of ridding the body of microorganisms, it serves the function of reprogramming cancerous cells.

How Antineoplastons Are Made

Most of the antineoplastons now being used are made synthetically from a patented manufacturing process; some are also produced from urine.

The methods used to make antineoplastons are highly complex and involve a series of integrated laboratory procedures. For example, antineoplaston A-10 is made by first acidifying a chemical solution isolated from urine. This acid is then heated for an extended duration and finally subjected to a multiple-step filtering process before it is administered to people.[6]

The High Cost of Antineoplaston Therapy

All patients who come to the Burzynski clinic are required to deposit $6,000 toward treatment costs. In some cases, patients may be charged an additional $3,000 per month beginning the second month of treatment.[7] These costs are generally out of pocket unless insurance companies reimburse the patient.*

Depending on the type of antineoplastons given, the costs may vary from $20 to $685 per day.[8] In addition, patients who require intravenous treatments outside of the clinic are required to purchase extra

---

*There are no absolute guidelines on the issue of coverage for alternative therapies. A therapy's standing within the medical community as well as an individual company's policy are variables which often influence the decision to reimburse patients.

supplies that can range from $80 to $5,000. On average, therapy can last from four months to one year.[9]

The BRI justifies its fees by citing the considerable expenses involved in developing and manufacturing antineoplastons. In addition, the BRI is described as a full-scale, state-of-the-art pharmaceutical facility that employs over 100 people, including a number of individuals holding doctorate degrees.

Dr. Burzynski claims that the cost of antineoplastons will drop considerably once the compounds are federally approved and marketed according to standard protocols.

Cancer Patients Who First Used Antineoplastons

In 1977, Dr. Burzynski treated twenty-one cancer patients with a peptide fraction he named "antineoplaston A."[10] According to a medical report, the patients all suffered from far advanced cancers including those of the breast, bladder, and colon.[11]

The cure rates and overall treatment results were tabulated as follows:

Effects	Number of Patients	Percentage of Total
Complete remission	4	19%
Partial remission	4	19
Stabilization of disease	6	28
Died	5	24
Discontinued treatment	2	10
TOTAL =	21	100%

Critics point out that this study represents Dr. Burzynski's observations and is not part of a large-scale, clinically controlled trial. However, if the Burzynski findings are scientifically accurate, then a total of 14 people either experienced complete remissions, partial remissions, or stabilization of their cancers as a result of antineoplaston therapy. Thus, a majority of the patients so treated could be said to have experienced improvement. Interestingly, of 1,248 patients treated with a standard chemotherapy regimen for the same types of cancers as those in the Burzynski group, only 2 achieved complete remissions; the overall total/partial remission rate was, in fact, only 4 percent.[12]

Other Studies Performed on Antineoplastons and the Scientific Communities' Reaction

Since Dr. Burzynski's 1977 clinical trial, he and other clinicians have performed a total of ninety studies on antineoplastons.[13] These studies were either published in peer-approved review journals or have appeared under the auspices of the BRI. The studies examine the effects of antineoplastons on animals, humans and tissue cultures.[14, 15]

In 1986, Burzynski was a featured speaker at the 14th International Cancer Congress—one of the most prestigious cancer research gatherings in the world.[16] He reported to his audience that a five-year follow-up of patients treated with antineoplastons showed the following:

—60 percent of patients experienced objective remission of their cancers

—47 percent obtained complete remissions

—20 percent survived beyond the five-year ceiling which commonly denotes a "cure"[17]

Eleven other published scientific papers supportive of antineoplastons were added as a supplement to the five-year trial.[18]

In 1991, Burzynski announced the results of another clinical trial of Antineoplaston 10 and a sister peptide fraction called Antineoplaston S2-1. In the study, one patient diagnosed with an advanced, terminal form of brain cancer went into complete remission and has remained disease-free.[19] The results of this report were submitted to the 17th International Congress of Chemotherapy, in Berlin, Germany.[20]

Other investigators both in the United States and abroad have also compiled evidence favorable to antineoplastons. In fact, dozens of positive reports exist, yet antineoplastons have been criticized and the ACS will not endorse their use.

According to Dr. Saul Green, who is a leading critic of antineoplastons, several factors seriously challenge the integrity of Burzynski and the entire premise of antineoplaston therapy. Following are the major criticisms against and the responses offered in defense of Dr. Burzynski and his claims:

1. *Antineoplastons are made from waste by-products that have no medicinal value.*

In an article appearing in the *Journal of the American Medical Association (JAMA)*, Green argued that antineoplastons break down into urinary waste products in the body.[21] In essence, Green is suggesting that people who are paying for a costly drug are simply receiving a useless substance with no therapeutic value.

Green also says that antineoplaston A-10 is insoluble in fluids and cannot be absorbed by bodily tissues. The entire premise of antineoplaston therapy, therefore, becomes suspect.

Response:

One of the "waste" by-products which make up antineoplastons has been found to actually block the growth of cancer cells[22] and interfere with abnormal cell division.[23, 24] Dr. Dvorit Samid and colleagues at the Uniformed Services University of Health Sciences, Bethesda, discovered that this by-product could actually help malignant cells establish normal patterns of growth.

According to a report appearing in the medical journal *Oncology News*, the by-product "can prevent [cancer] formation and suppress the growth of malignant cells carrying [faulty cancer] genes."[25] Dr. Samid stated that "such a dramatic phenomenon is seldom seen...I am very excited about these findings."[26]

Speaking before the 9th International Symposium on Future Trends in Chemotherapy, the Bethesda scientist concluded that antineoplastons

> have a direct antitumor activity...not killing [the cancer cell] but making it behave more normally...because [antineoplastons] are natural compounds, the body tolerates them well, and therefore, we minimize the problem of adverse effects. Antineoplastons could be a very valuable, effective, and safe approach to cancer therapy.[27]

Interestingly, Dr. Samid's findings were published six months *after* Dr. Green wrote his critical article in *JAMA*.[28] When questioned, Dr.

Green admitted that this discrepancy was the obvious reason he did not quote Dr. Samid's work.[29]

Regarding the issue of solubility, Burzynski proponents maintain that antineoplastons are "more soluble" than common proteins obtained in most healthy diets.[30] Japanese scientists have also verified this conclusion.[31]

2. Antineoplaston research is not being supported by independent scientists as the Burzynski Institute claims.

According to an informational brochure supplied by the BRI, scientists in Japan and other countries planned to "conduct clinical trials" with antineoplastons on a variety of tumors including those of the brain, blood, prostate, and breast.[32, 33] But in later correspondence, officials allegedly denied having shown any interest in Dr. Burzynski's methods.

For example, the president of the National Cancer Center in Tokyo told Dr. Green that: "I am afraid. . . . antineoplaston[s] [have] no popularity in our country."[34] Further, the chief Japanese researcher involved in the study said:

> we do not think that you arc going to pick up any biological effect of antineoplaston A-10 in our study.[35]

Response:

In a rebuttal, Dr. Burzynski argued that the researcher's comments were taken completely out of context. For example, the statement that Dr. Green would not "pick up any" anticancer activity from antineoplastons was, according to the Japanese researcher who made it, a misquote. According to a follow-up letter by the researcher, his original point was that Dr. Green—not being an M.D.—would not have had "sufficient" "qualifications" to evaluate the Japanese studies.[36] In fact, the Japanese researcher verified that antineoplastons did inhibit "human breast cancer remarkably in 2–3 weeks."[37]

Japanese scientists also found that antineoplastons could prevent tumor formation and block the deadly spread of liver cancers.[38]

3. National Cancer Institute studies have failed to show any anticancer effects in animals from antineoplastons.

The NCI's first animal study on antineoplastons was negative and is considered crucial by some observers, because it has influenced much of the later criticisms over antineoplastons.

Response:
Dr. Burzynski has long maintained that his treatment affects animals far differently than it does humans. Japanese researchers also found test "discrepancies" between animals and humans[39] that could be corrected by giving the right amounts of antineoplastons.[40]

The NCI's first failed study has thus been blamed on an incorrectly used dosage of antineoplastons. As a matter of record, Dr. Burzynski had warned investigators prior to the study that he did not "believe [his] compound [would] display [anticancer] activity" when used on animals.[41] However, a third series of tests were performed at a "correct dosage" on the proper animal model and antitumor activity was reported.[42]

Despite the conflicts surrounding NCI's first unsuccessful test, a number of other animal studies have shown favorable results. For example, in two separate experiments published by Chinese scientists and independent researchers in the United States, antineoplastons were definitely found to inhibit tumors.[43, 44]

4. *Antineoplastons have not shown any effect against cancer in humans*
According to the American Cancer Society's most recent fact sheet on Burzynski, antineoplastons are not

fit for administration to humans, and...there is no reason to believe that Dr. Burzynski has discovered an effective cure for cancer.[45]

The ACS also points out that researchers found "inadequate scientific evidence to justify the use of antineoplastons" in humans.[46] In addition, NCI scientists found "no anticancer activity" in a review of seven people with brain cancer, according to the agency.[47]

Response:
There are a number of contradictions in the ACS fact sheet on

antineoplastons. For example, a footnote was added to the critique which reads:

> In March 1989, the FDA acted on a request from Dr. Burzynski and his colleagues to conduct a small clinical trial on anti-neoplaston therapy in the treatment of advanced... breast cancer. The FDA has granted permission for this clinical trial to proceed under the Investigational New Drug guidelines. This will be the first independently monitored evaluation of antineoplaston therapy in human beings.[48]

According to an article appearing in an insurance industry journal, the FDA conducted a site visit to Japan in 1989 and found "important animal studies [were being] done confirming Dr. Burzynski's work."[49] Also, in a letter written by the Antineoplaston Study Group at the Kurume Medical School, the Japanese commented that "we believe... the FDA inspectors had a good impression of our study."[50]

During the time that the denunciatory ACS report appeared, additional studies supporting the positive effects of antineoplastons had emerged.

In 1991, for instance, a Phase II clinical trial of twenty patients with brain malignancies treated with antineoplastons revealed that 25 percent attained complete remissions, 10 percent partial remissions and 50 percent "objective stabilization" of their cancers (objective stabilization means that disease progression has ceased although the patient may still have evidence of cancer).[51]

In another study, a group of men suffering from prostate cancer were treated with a combination of antineoplastons and hormones. In that trial, 2 patients experienced complete remission, 3 partial remissions, and 7, objective stabilization of their cancers.[52]

In wake of this new evidence, the NCI reversed its earlier negative findings on antineoplastons. According to the institute's associate director of the Developmental Therapeutics Program, antineoplastons have definitely demonstrated anticancer activity.[53]

Because Dr. Green wrote his critique *before* the NCI reached its new conclusions, he did not yet have the benefit of data to materialize. Indeed, it was at the end of Green's article that *JAMA* appended the following footnote:

Since the manuscript [Green's] was accepted for publication, the NCI announced that on October 4, 1991, NCI site-visit team headed by M. J. Hawkings M.D., visited the Burzynski Research Institute, where they reviewed a best-case series of seven patients prepared for them by Burzynski. . . . based on their review, the NCI had decided to conduct four independent Phase II clinical trials on patients with [specific forms of brain cancer] using antineoplastons A-10 and AS2-1.[54]

In July 1993, an IND (Investigation of New Drug) permit passed final clearance, and the NCI began to move forward with its testing of antineoplastons.[55]

Dr. Burzynski's Ongoing Legal Disputes

In 1983, a suit was launched against Dr. Burzynski by the FDA for using an unapproved drug. But a U.S. District Court Judge ruled that federal law did not prohibit the researcher from treating patients in Texas.[56] Two years later, FDA agents and federal marshals conducted a raid on BRI and reportedly seized a number of confidential files; the files were being held for a number of years despite attempts by Burzynski and supportive patients to reclaim them.[57]

In 1986, the Aetna Insurance Company initiated a racketeering suit against Burzynski, charging him with conspiracy to defraud them by using an unproven, expensive treatment. Burzynski lawyers launched a countersuit charging Aetna with conspiracy to put BRI out of business.[58] Interestingly, if the NCI proves that antineoplastons do have anticancer activity in humans, it could mean an end to Aetna's allegations and the beginning of that company's defense against a potentially large countersuit.

Currently, the Texas Department of Health has cited the BRI with four violations. This latest suit alleges that Burzynski is unjustified in treating people with an unapproved drug. As in the past, patients who claim to have been helped by antineoplaston treatment have begun a crusade to defend what they consider unfair and vicious persecution of a humanitarian physician and an effective and safe cancer treatment.

Ironically, this latest in a long series of attempts to shut down the Burzynski clinic comes at the very time the NCI had admitted finding merit with the controversial cancer therapy.

Unlike many unorthodox cancer practitioners, Dr. Burzynski has been affiliated with a number of highly regarded medical institutions, has shared his treatment concepts before prestigious scientific gatherings throughout the world, has repeatedly petitioned government agencies to test his compounds, and has published his theories and research results extensively in accredited medical journals, fulfilling the standards considered sine qua non among scientists. Considering that one of the most common criticisms leveled at alternative cancer physicians is the *lack* of published data concerning their concepts and treatment methods, Burzynski's credentials stand up.

Regarding the actual merit of antineoplastons, a number of published studies do suggest that they work against certain types of cancers. In some cases, cures have been documented and a number of these are a matter of medical and court record.

Is antineoplaston therapy a cure for cancer? In a recent interview, cancer historian Ralph Moss commented:

I don't know if it's a cure. Unlike most other nontoxic cancer treatments, [antineoplastons do] shrink tumors. The NCI team that made the site visit to Burzynski's Institute could see this from the CAT scans.[59]

If antineoplastons have shown such positive anticancer effects, why does division between mainstream researchers and Burzynski advocates remain?

Some scientists refute the concept of antineoplaston therapy, based on Dr. Burzynski's peptide theory, which at this time has not received a consensus of scientific support. Yet, certain chemicals in antineoplastons have, in fact, shown powerful effects against cancer cells—whatever the ultimate fate of the peptide theory.

Regardless of the scientific debate that has evolved over the years, preliminary evidence appears to be favoring antineoplastons as a potentially new alternative in nontoxic cancer treatment. Indeed, both the NCI and FDA are moving ahead with a clinical trial after reviewing patients with terminal brain cancer; it would be unlikely for those agencies to approve clinical testing of a drug not shown to have any benefits in preliminary screening.

Until all the data are in, however, antineoplastons will remain an "unproven" treatment for cancer and will continue to be frowned on by the ACS and, undoubtedly, the majority of practicing U.S. physicians. And even if antineoplastons do become accepted by the mainstream, they may not prove to be a universal cancer remedy; thus far, the best treatment results in humans have involved cancers of the brain and prostate.

Those considering antineoplaston therapy should carefully review all the available facts and the track record of the drug regarding specific types of cancers. Moreover, patients should receive written confirmation from their insurance carriers that treatment is covered. In a number of cases, insurance companies have been warned by the FDA of potential illegality for endorsing payment of antineoplastons because of their "unproven" status.[60]

For further information contact:

Burzynski Clinic
6221 Corporate Drive
Houston, TX 77036
(713) 777-8233

NINE

Hyperthermia

While not commonly associated with traditional cancer therapy, hyperthermia—which is the use of heat to kill cancer cells—has become accepted within mainstream medicine. Yet this modality of treatment still is not commonly applied, nor is it well known to the general public.

Hyperthermia was first practiced thousands of years ago by the ancient Egyptians. Hippocrates, the "father" of modern medicine, also dabbled in the treatment. Through the centuries, physicians realized that heat had a telling effect on tumors and, in some cases, could even cause their remission. This realization prompted Dr. William Bradford Coley's therapeutic use of infectious organisms to stimulate fever in his patients as a means of treating cancer early this century.

During the 1960s, researchers verified that cancer cells are, in fact, much more sensitive to heat than their normal counterparts.[1] Moreover, heat has also been shown to stimulate the immune system's cancer-fighting ability by helping the body manufacture interferon—a crucial immunity protein.

In its current form, hyperthermia is applied in a number of ways. For example, plastic or fiber-optic cylinders may be inserted directly into tumors and used to deliver ultrasound or microwave heat energy to malignant cells. Other techniques involve the implanting of magnetic rods into malignant tissues, which are then heated. Sapphire probes are also used, and these can deliver bursts of laser-generated heat that is destructive to malignant cells.

Because many of these techniques cause more destruction to the inner core of tumors but not the outer edges, some researchers feel that hyperthermia is more effective when used conjunctively with other therapies such as radiation or chemotherapy.

Hyperthermia's Effectiveness According to the Most Recent Studies

A number of clinicians are reporting moderate to highly effective results with hyperthermia for some types of otherwise incurable cancers.

In one study, for example, seven patients with metastatic brain cancer were treated with a hyperthermia implant device. After treatment, researchers noted two "complete responses" and one minor response. They concluded that "hyperthermia...is a very useful and promising method for treating" brain cancer.[2]

In another study, probes were used to administer laser-generated heat into liver tumors, and afterward physicians found evidence of necrosis (i.e., cell death) of the tumors. They concluded that "selective destruction of malignant liver tumors is possible with...laser induced hyperthermia."[3]

Further positive results were noted with usually intractable and incurable cancers of the liver, pancreas, and bone. When a team of Japanese scientists introduced a warmed drug solution into blood vessels feeding the tumors, a remarkable 73 percent response rate was noted.[4]

A similar technique was used on 31 patients with stomach cancer but in this case, a warmed solution was perfused (i.e. poured) in and around the abdominal cavity immediately after surgery. This procedure resulted in the survival of 82 percent of the heat-treated patients for one year, compared with only 40 percent in the untreated, control group; after three years, 26 percent of the hyperthermia-treated patients were still alive, while *all* of the controls had died.[5]

The Effectiveness of Hyperthermia Combined With Traditional Cancer Treatment

Hyperthermia has been shown to increase the susceptibility of cancer cell membranes to standard drug therapies.[6] In addition, researchers have found that hyperthermia may increase the cancer-killing capability of radiation therapy threefold.[7] In fact, better responses have been noted with this combined approach than from radiation alone.[8]

In one study involving recurring chest cancers, for example, hyperthermia and radiation resulted in 83 percent remission rates for early stage disease and 25 percent remission in advanced cases.[9]

In another study, researchers treated twenty-five seriously ill kidney cancer patients with a combination of hyperthermia, radiation, and chemotherapy. This treatment resulted in "an immediate stabilization of the health" of all the patients—including some partial or total regressions.[10] Such a finding is particularly noteworthy since late stage kidney tumors are especially difficult to treat and none of the traditional methods have thus far proved successful.

The American Cancer Society's View of Hyperthermia

Although dozens of corroborative studies have appeared in the peer-review literature since the turn of the century, the ACS did not remove hyperthermia from its *Unproven List* until 1977. While the agency supports its use in cancer treatment currently hyperthermia still is not considered a primary treatment modality.

Since 1977, an estimated 10,000 people have been treated with hyperthermia in the United States.

Dangers Associated With Hyperthermia

Hyperthermia may not be completely safe because misdirected heat can destroy healthy tissues. However, the treatment is considered generally nontoxic when performed by knowledgeable physicians.

Hyperthermia is a viable treatment option for a number of different cancers; it has also been shown to enhance the cancer-killing effects of standard therapies. In some cases, it is considered superior to chemotherapy.[11]

Interestingly, hyperthermia may offer potentially life-saving benefits not offered by toxic therapies. For example, in cancers that may be inaccessible and untreatable, such as those affecting the pancreas, liver, or parts of the brain, heat therapies (usually in combination with other methods) have had remarkable effects—at least in preliminary studies. As researchers develop better techniques to deliver heat energy to specific malignant "targets," response ratios will undoubtedly improve.

Those interested in hyperthermia as an adjunct to traditional therapy should screen hyperthermia clinics that specialize in multi-combinational approaches or are affiliated with other centers that do. Also, current trends in hyperthermia and its usefulness regarding specific forms of cancer should be carefully investigated.

For further information contact:

Valley Cancer Institute
12099 West Washington Blvd., Suite 304
Los Angeles, CA 90066
(310) 398-0013

TEN

Hoxsey Method

The Hoxsey method ranks among the most colorful, if not maligned twentieth-century alternative cancer methods on record. Its developer, Harry Hoxsey, was considered a quack of the highest magnitude, but recent scientific research has partly corroborated the anticancer activity of his medicines.

The original Hoxsey treatment consisted of an ointment or "escharotic" salve used on external cancers. Later, Hoxsey formulated a "tonic" for internal malignancies. After Hoxsey divulged the ingredients of his "secret" formula during a Food and Drug Administration (FDA) investigation in the 1950s, a number of studies on the formula's components were conducted. These studies were done under the auspices of government agencies who had shown a long-standing antagonism toward Hoxsey's "quack" remedies.

Armed with the results of its investigations, the American Cancer Society (ACS) and the FDA presented evidence (during the course of three federal trials) that the Hoxsey medicines were completely "worthless."[1] However, a number of loyal patients persisted in maintaining Hoxsey's credibility and to this day, the method continues to be used yearly by hundreds of people, many of whom have reported being "cured."

Ironically, Harry Hoxsey died from prostate cancer in 1973. His treatment is now offered at the Bio-Medical Center in Tijuana under the direction of Mildred Nelson, a nurse who formerly worked for Hoxsey.

Hoxsey's Credentials

Hoxsey reportedly did not have any formal education in the sciences. His purported knowledge of cancer treatment was based on information passed down from his great-grandfather, who first devised the herbal salve.

During Hoxsey's life, he became wealthy through investments in oil and, according to the ACS, through his many cancer clinics.

A large-scale, scientific trial of Hoxsey's treatment has never been conducted. However, the ACS as well as the FDA did review the records of patients who had claimed favorable results after receiving the controversial remedy. According to the ACS, it is virtually impossible to attach significance to these favorable claims because 90 percent of the patients received conventional therapies before embarking on the Hoxsey program.[2] In addition, an FDA review of 400 patients was said to show a "consistent pattern" which reinforced the worthlessness of Hoxsey's therapy. For example, a number of the 400 patients were found not to have had cancer in the first place; another group had proven cancer but were "successfully" treated by previous means. Another sampling of patients still had evidence of cancer, which progressed to death despite Hoxsey's treatment.[3] Further, the ACS states that a "carefully" controlled experiment using Hoxsey's medicine on mice showed no appreciable reduction in the size of tumors.[4]

Official Studies of Hoxsey's Medicines

According to a government analysis, the "primary ingredient" of the Hoxsey formula is potassium iodide, which was used many years ago to treat tumor-like conditions resulting from syphilis. Potassium iodide was then tried on cancer but later abandoned after it was found to possess no benefits.

The tonics also contain licorice and pepsin, which only serve as "flavorings." Cascara, buckthorn bark, and stillingia root are considered to have only "laxative" properties. Other ingredients include red clover ("discredited" as an antivenereal herb in 1912), burdock root (now "obsolete"), berberis root (which is only of "historical interest"), and pokeweed, which can cause "severe illness requiring hospitalization."[5]

The ACS thus concluded that Hoxsey medicines are "both useless" when used internally, and "archaic" when applied externally.[6]

Studies Contradicting the ACS

While there are no data supporting or refuting the Hoxsey therapy in terms of large-scale, scientifically controlled human trials, recent studies do corroborate the anticancer effects of the therapy's ingredients. For example, buckthorn, which is said to be only a laxative, has been found to contain a tumor-inhibiting factor that has shown activity against leukemia. Japanese scientists also isolated a crucial substance from burdock which inhibits cellular mutation, a key factor in the cancer process.[7] And investigators have isolated antitumor properties in berberis.[8]

Intriguingly, while the ACS argues that pokeweed can cause severe illness and is not therapeutically useful for anything,[9] a growing body of research indicates that this herb may play a useful role in cancer treatment, detection, and augmentation of the immune system. In fact, pokeweed has become an important subject of research in a number of mainstream cancer labaratories throughout the world.

As a diagnostic tool, scientists have found that antibody-like proteins from pokeweed show an affinity for malignant cells—specifically those affecting the colon; in this regard, pokeweed proteins may prove useful for diagnosing malignant colon cancers.[10]

From a *treatment* standpoint, pokeweed has been shown to stimulate the synthesis of interleukins—the much-touted protein factors crucial to immunity and the control of cancer.[11]

Besides influencing the production of interleukins, pokeweed is also involved in the reproduction and growth of T and B cells—both of which are critical to immune-system functioning.[12] Perhaps the most significant finding to date has been that pokeweed contains special types of molecules known as *mitogens*; mitogens have been shown to *regulate* the division of cells—a factor which is missing in the cancer process.[13]

While these reports do not validate the Hoxsey therapy, they offer surprising new evidence of anticancer activity by some of the individual ingredients. At the very least, the claim that Hoxsey's medicines are without any merit whatsoever does not bear the weight of current scientific analysis.

The Hoxsey Clinic and the Cost for Treatment

At present, the Bio-Medical Center in Tijuana, Mexico, offers a program including a physical examination, X-rays, CAT-scans, and blood work.[14]. Tonics and escharotic medicines are given as deemed necessary and provided as long as patients need them. In addition to Hoxsey medicines, the Bio-Medical Center employs vitamins, minerals and other "nontoxic" substances; a diet is also implemented which restricts pork, tomatoes, alcohol, salt, sugar, and other foods.

The fee for treatment is $3,500 and this includes a lifetime supply of medication. The cost for tests are additional.

A Recent Documentary on Hoxsey and His Treatment

Hoxsey: When Healing Becomes a Crime, was produced by independent filmmakers and premiered in September 1987 at the Margaret Mead Film Festival in New York City.

The film, which examines the politics and suppression of the much-touted Hoxsey remedy, aired on cable television and is now also on video.

While the ACS claims the Hoxsey remedy is worthless, recent scientific studies have shown that the formula's herbs possess a range of immune-stimulating and cell-regulating characteristics. Pokeweed has received much of the attention and is now being considered for use as a diagnostic tool in some cancers as well as a powerful immune-system booster.

These findings do not necessarily translate into therapeutic benefit for people with cancer. But they do suggest that the herbs used in the Hoxsey formula may prove valuable as part of a comprehensive, holistic cancer-treatment program. In fact, some patients use Hoxsey herbs in conjunction with orthodox cancer treatments.

At this time, the only clinical "evidence" of benefit from the Hoxsey treatment remains testimonial case histories. Interested persons are thus urged to contact and review, whenever possible, the medical records of formerly treated patients according to the type and location of cancer.

Several distributors in the United States offer herbal preparations similar to those in the Hoxsey medicines; these may provide a cheaper alternative for patients. However, because pokeweed is a potentially poisonous plant, it should be used with caution and only under the supervision of a health professional or qualified herbalist experienced in its use.

For further information contact:

On Hoxsey treatment:

Bio-Medical Center
P.O. Box 727
General Ferreira #615
Colonia Juarez,
Tijuana, B.C.
Mexico 22000
011 52 66-84-90-11
011 52 66-84-90-81
011 52 66-84-90-82

On herbal preparations:

Eclectic Institute
11231 S.E. Market Street
Portland, OR 97216
1 (800) 332-4372

On pokeweed preparations*:

The International Herb Brokers
Apopka, FL
1 (407) 869-9979

On Hoxsey video:

Order from Cancer Control Society
(see Appendix). Film lasts 1 hour,
36 minutes and is priced at $36.

*Also check your local telephone directory under "herbs."

ELEVEN

Oxygen Therapies

Oxygen therapy, used in the management of cancer, is sometimes also called "hyperoxygenation," "oxymedicine," or "bio-oxidative" therapy.

Oxygen treatments take on a number of different forms. For example, patients may be given solutions of hydrogen peroxide (which breaks down into oxygen in the blood) or they might receive infusions of ozone gas. In some cases, vitamins and minerals that are supposed to increase the oxygenation of the blood and tissues (for example vitamin E, germanium, and Coenzyme Q) may also be used supplementally.

The premise of oxygen therapy is that "toxic" conditions in the body which lead to disease are caused by a lowered concentration of oxygen in the cells and tissues. Holistic physicians believe that by increasing the oxygen concentration in diseased tissues and blood, the body's toxicity can be reversed and illnesses—including cancer—can be cured. Some physicians also believe that cancer cells thrive in anaerobic (without oxygen) conditions and are thus adversely affected by hyperoxygenating treatments. Further, oxygenation procedures are believed to promote unstable but beneficial molecules that act as "scavengers" of harmful free radicals linked to the cancer process.

Currently, the American Cancer Society (ACS) considers oxygen treatments without merit and argues that the "claims made for oxymedicine far exceed any demonstrated efficacy."[1]

Hydrogen Peroxide in Medicine

During the 1918 influenza epidemic, physicians claimed to have reduced a number of fatalities with hydrogen peroxide (abbreviated "H_2O_2"). In the 1950s and 1960s, scientists also began to explore other disease-treatment possibilities with the chemical. Since that time, a sizable number of people have taken hydrogen peroxide intravenously and orally—although this last method is considered unsafe by a number of practitioners.

The Benefits of Hydrogen Peroxide Use in Cancer Treatment

According to Dr. Charles H. Farr, a leading proponent of oxygen therapy, many bodily conditions unfavorable to cancer are created by hydrogen peroxide, including an increase in the metabolic rate and a raised temperature. Farr also believes that hydrogen peroxide attacks harmful free radicals and is destructive to viruses, bacteria and other organisms—some of which may act as co-factors in the malignant process. In addition, studies have shown that hydrogen peroxide does work against cancer directly.[2]

Dangers of Hydrogen Peroxide Use

Critics argue that hydrogen peroxide can react with free radicals in the body causing a range of problems, from gout to aging.[3] Others cite experiments in which animals died after being given the drug.[4] But Dr. Farr insists that no major studies show injury to humans. Further, the extensive use of H_2O_2 and the disproportionate absence of side effects is seen as proof regarding safety. Farr also says that H_2O_2 is naturally produced in the body and that it serves a host of vital functions; his claim has been corroborated by Professor B. Halliwell of the Department of Biochemistry, University of London.

Some researchers suggest that dangerous free radicals resulting from overuse of H_2O_2 can be neutralized by taking supplements of an enzyme known as *superoxide dismutase* (SOD). SOD is found in the body and serves a valuable role by converting dangerous free radicals into less harmful constituents.[5]

The Rationale for Using Ozone in Cancer Treatment

Like hydrogen peroxide, ozone's oxygenating properties are believed to help reverse the airless conditions favorable to some cancers. The gas is also believed to create unstable molecules which scavenge viruses, bacteria, and other microorganisms possibly affecting cancer patients.[6]

Physicians began using ozone (abbreviated "O_3") in 1915 to speed up wound healing and, later, to treat such diseases as ulcerative colitis.[7]

Ozone's Efficacy in Cancer Treatment

While most of the human trials conducted on ozone have not been scientifically controlled, some studies do show benefits. In one experiment, test doses of ozone effectively inhibited cancer-cell division; the greater the doses, the more inhibition occurred, reaching almost complete cessation of cancer-cell activity.[8] In another study, ozone was shown to enhance the tumor-fighting ability of standard cancer drugs.[9]

Researchers from the Institute of General Physiology and Nutritional Sciences in Italy also found that ozone treatments appear to activate the immune system by stimulating production of potent cancer-killing proteins known as *cytokines*.[10] The researchers concluded that ozone's "large range of medical applications...could become very valuable" in cancer treatment.[11]

Although the ACS officially disputes ozone's therapeutic value, it does mention several positive cancer studies. According to the ACS:

> Well-designed studies by two research teams have found that a variety of tumor cell types exposed to ozone in vitro were more susceptible than healthy cells to damage and destruction. Both groups suggest possible mechanisms and state that they believe further research is indicated.[12]

Other Applications of Ozone Therapy

A number of recent experiments suggest that ozone can benefit other medical conditions besides cancer. For example, an ozone solution used to irrigate dangerous abdominal abscesses improved the condition of test animals substantially.[13] In another study involving oxygen deprivation, ozone treatment helped to restore a normal degree of brain function and also prolonged survival time in animals.[14] In humans, a number of impressive results have also been noted.

Injections of ozone significantly improved circulation-related problems in the extremities of heart patients.[15] In addition, transfusions of the gas were found to help a number of eye diseases, ranging from glaucoma to optic neuritis.[16]

Currently, ozone is used to treat a wide range of illnesses including candidiasis, AIDS, hepatitis, diabetes, and artery disease.

How Ozone is Administered

Various methods are used. In one treatment known as *auto-hemotherapy*, 50 to 100 milliliters of blood are drawn, mixed with a purified ozone/oxygen mixture, and then re-injected into the patient. Other techniques involve injecting ozone into muscle tissues or administering it orally; this last strategy is sometimes used to treat gastric cancers.

Dangers Associated with Ozone Therapy

Some data suggest that ozone can, under certain conditions, cause potential danger. Scientists found that "depending on the extent of duration" to O_3 exposure, experimental mice could develop problems in metabolizing proteins, with resultant damage to their hearts.[17] (Note that this report is in contrast to the one cited earlier involving heart patients).

In another study, hamsters exposed to ozone did not develop any more respiratory problems or cancers than control animals, contrary to popular suspicions about these untold effects.[18]

Oxygen therapy advocates point out that the dangerous effects commonly associated with ozone are *not* from therapeutic doses of the gas and are often confused with *ozone pollution*; this phenomenon occurs when ozone (which in its pure form is vital to the protection of earth's atmosphere from ultraviolet radiation) interacts with smog and other pollutants to form a dangerous environmental hazard.

Oxygen therapies are not generally considered a sole treatment of choice for cancer. For this reason, a number of holistic and metabolic clinicians use oxymedicine as an adjunct to other therapies. The Gerson clinic, for example, supplements its usual diet method with ozone, when indicated.

Controversy over safety is still an issue, but oxygen treatments have been given to thousands of people without ill effects. In some cases, potential problems, including free-radical damage, may occur, but these are usually linked to improper use; clinicians thus speak of a "therapeutic window" of safety that should not exceed recommended treatment doses.

People considering oxygen therapies should only consult a medical doctor who has had lengthy experience in their use.

For further information contact:

On hydrogen peroxide:

Michael B. Schachter, M.D.
Two Executive Blvd., Suite 202
Suffern, NY 10901
(914) 368-4727

American Metabolic Institute
524 Calle Primera Road, Suite 1005A
San Ysidro, CA 92173
(619) 229-3003
1 (800) 388-1083

On ozone:

Ahmed Elkadi, M.D.
Akbar Clinic
236 South Tyndall Parkway
Panama City, FL 32404
(904) 763-7689

T W E L V E

Iscador

Iscador, a controversial cancer drug made from the mistletoe plant, was first proposed as a treatment for cancer in 1920 by Rudolf Steiner. Steiner, who was a biologist and philosopher, founded the Society for Cancer Research in Arlesheim, Switzerland. Since Iscador was first used in 1921, a number of successes against cancer have been reported.

Although Iscador is a drug, Steiner's rationale for using it was based on philosophical considerations. In Steiner's view, mistletoe, like the cancer cell, defies nature by its wild growth and adherence to its own natural rhythms (for example, flowering in the winter). Yet, this seeming lack of orderliness is overshadowed by the plant's ability to grow, bear fruit, and follow a well-organized pattern of development or, in biological terms, *differentiation*. Based on this premise, Steiner theorized that mistletoe could also impart a sense of order and balance to renegade cancer cells in the body.

There was more to Steiner's proposed cancer treatment than just mistletoe. Drawing on earlier philosophies, Steiner developed a belief-system known as *anthroposophy* whereby healing came to be viewed as a process involving mind, body, and spirit.[1] In this sense, cancer could be better managed by channeling the life-giving "forces" of the mind into the physical body. Conversely, negative, unhappy emotions could cause a disruption in the life-giving forces, and this could lead to cancer.

While remaining silent on the premise of anthroposophy in the treatment of disease, the American Cancer Society (ACS) disputes claims of benefit for Iscador and has prohibited its use in the United States. At this time, however, the drug has been approved in a number of European countries including Germany, where 15,000 physicians are said to be using mistletoe preparations in treatment.

The Leading Proponent of Iscador Therapy

Dr. Rita Leroi, a supervisor at the Lukas clinic in Arlesheim, Switzerland, is currently the foremost supporter of Iscador therapy.

Keeping in the anthroposophical tradition, Dr. Leroi combines Iscador with psychological enhancing techniques such as insight therapy, to help patients dispel negative emotions and increase the positive "spiritual" forces believed to play crucial roles in healing. She also employs music and motion therapies (to help address the physical/spiritual needs of the patient) and prescribes a vegetarian diet.

Studies that Corroborate Iscador's Alleged Benefits

A number of scientific papers and monographs that support Iscador's "tumor-fighting" ability have been published since Steiner's death. In addition, both the Lukas clinic and the Ludvig Boltzmann Institute in Austria have conducted over forty clinical studies on the drug, and many positive benefits—including cures—have been reported. The studies were criticized, however, for being poorly organized.[2]

The American Cancer Society's Findings on Iscador

The ACS disputes Iscador after a review of "17 clinical and chemical papers" was conducted by "two expert consultants." The consultants also reviewed an additional 25 papers and 14 unpublished manuscripts on the drug and saw little in these papers to change their negative opinion.[3]

The ACS thus concludes that no evidence exists favoring Iscador for "the treatment of cancer in humans." But in its report, the ACS admits that published studies do show mistletoe stimulates thymus-gland activity (crucial to immunity) and also "speed up the regeneration of blood-forming cells after exposure to X-rays" (advocates have long touted Iscador's reported benefits for patients undergoing radiation therapy).

The ACS also mentions that potent alkaloids from European Iscador were found to inhibit human leukemia cells in the test tube.[4]

The ACS Criticism of Iscador

According to medical historian Robert Houston, one of the reviewing consultants in the ACS denunciation was an "outspoken opponent" of unorthodox therapies, even chairing a committee to expose them; the second consultant was a pioneer of orthodox chemotherapy, having "gone on record" as opposing alternative cancer medicine.[5] Houston and other critics thus question the objectivity and impartiality of such established opponents of alternative cancer therapies.

Another problem with the ACS review (conducted prior to 1982), is that it does not take into account the number of studies performed *after* 1982 which lend support to mistletoe's tumor-fighting properties.

In 1993, for example, German researchers reported that a mistletoe lectin (antibody-like protein found in plants) has a powerful immune-modulating effect on white blood cells crucial to immunity.[6]

In another recent study, mistletoe was found to reduce the occurrence of a potentially dangerous blood condition known as *leukopenia*; this abnormality—which generally results from exposure to cancer drugs or radiation—was favorably controlled in animals receiving a combination of drugs, radiation, and mistletoe extract.[7] Researchers concluded that mistletoe could be used along with chemotherapy and radiation therapy.[8]

Scientists from the Institute of General Physiology and Nutritional Science at Siena, Italy, also suggested that mistletoe could be useful as an adjuvant in the biological therapy of cancer. The Italian investigators, upon clarifying that mistletoe acts as a powerful inflammatory mediator able to stimulate the immune system, emphasized that the drug should not be ignored any longer.[9]

Not all research on Iscador has been limited to its effects on immunity. Several studies have shown, for example, that the drug could extend survival time in humans afflicted with varying degrees of cancer. Conversely, a few trials involving advanced cancer patients showed ambiguous or negative results.

While the therapeutic benefits of Iscador remain a subject of controversy in the United States, European clinicians routinely use the drug, usually in combination with other treatment modalities.

At this time, current opinion holds that Iscador is more useful against solid tumors; cancers of the blood and blood-forming organs are considered less responsive to therapy. Recent scientific research also corroborates Iscador's potential for reducing dangerous side effects associated with chemotherapy and radiation. In this regard, the drug may serve as a useful adjuvant to more traditional cancer therapies.

Despite the ACS stance against Iscador, a number of scientists are beginning to take it seriously. Indeed, the researchers who had criticized Dr. Leroi's studies for being poorly organized admitted that in view of their own "positive experiences," Iscador should be subjected to a "randomized multicenter study" for further evaluation.[10]

Issues of safety have been raised, but Iscador appears to be relatively nontoxic when used by experienced clinicians. However, mistletoe—from which Iscador is derived—can be poisonous, and its leaves or berries should never be eaten.

Those contemplating Iscador in the treatment of cancer should do so only under expert supervision and at established clinics.

For further information contact:

Hufeland Klinik for Holistic Immunotherapy
D-6990 Bad Mergentheim
Germany
011 49-7931-7082

Lukas Klinik
CH-4144 Arlesheim
Switzerland
011 41-61-72-3333

THIRTEEN

Live Cell Therapy

Live cell therapy (also known as "fresh cell" or "cellular therapy") was developed by the Swiss physician Paul Niehans in 1931. Beside being a medical doctor, Neihans also earned doctoral degrees in science, medical philosophy, and theology.

Niehans claimed that after a patient who lacked a parathyroid gland was treated with living cells from a calf's parathyroid, the patient's own gland grew back.[1] Based on this bizarre finding, Niehans theorized that living cells have a capacity for bonding with similar cells and regenerating them. According to this concept, liver cells will be attracted to the liver, heart cells to the heart, brain cells to the brain, and so on. Neihans proposed that injections of living, healthy embryonic cells from young animals could be used to "target" and heal diseased organs and tissues in people. The physician first attempted to cure diabetes and glandular abnormalities and later focused on other illnesses. After treating 5,000 patients, Neihans published a book detailing his "successes" with live cell therapy.[2]

Overall, 60,000 people have been treated with live cells since the 1930s for a variety of conditions. The most famous of these include Pope Pius XII, Somerset Maugham, and Pablo Picasso.[3]

Following up on Niehan's research, German scientists began administering live umbilical-cord cells to cancer patients, theorizing that these would regenerate the immune system to fight tumors. Highly beneficial results were reported following these treatments, including cures and remissions.

The American Cancer Society (ACS) disputes these reports, arguing that they consist only of "select case histories" and are not scientifically founded. Further, a number of dangerous side effects have been linked to live cell therapy, and for this reason, the ACS advises that people not seek this form of treatment.[4]

Research Supporting the Rationale Behind Live Cell Therapy

A number of favorable scientific studies have been conducted, primarily in animals. In one experiment, cells from the hormone-producing glands of a hamster were given to a rat, and this led to increased production of hormones from the rat's own cells.[5] In another study, scientists from the University of Heidelberg "tagged" live cells with radioactive isotopes. When these were injected into host animals, the tagged cells were found to be "transported" to their counterpart cells in the host.[6]

Dr. A. Kment of the University of Vienna Veterinary College discovered that live cell injections could also rejuvenate tissues of the nervous system; this, in turn, improved learning skills in test animals.[7] In yet another intriguing experiment, living spleen cells from rats and fetal cells from sheep prevented other animals from developing chemically induced tumors.[8]

In the realm of human cancer treatment, Dr. Wolfram Kuhnau (a leading disciple of Dr. Niehans) claims to have cured a number of people who had exhausted the hope of all other therapies. Kuhnau cites one patient with progressing liver cancer who went into complete remission after live cell injections. In another case, a boy with advanced bone cancer also experienced a total regression after treatment.[9]

Dr. Kuhnau points out that cellular therapies are not considered a single treatment for cancer but are generally used in combination with other strategies.

How Live Cells Are Used in Cancer Therapy

Fetal cells from young animals are generally used to treat cancer—as well as other diseases. These cells are preferred because immunity is not fully developed in embryonic tissues, and thus the risk of "rejection" in humans is supposedly reduced.

Dr. Kuhnau believes that malignant tumors are an outgrowth of underlying metabolic disturbances in the body. In his view, the forces which perpetuate tumor growth must be corrected by stimulating immunity and "balancing" the hormonal system. This correction should take place early in a patient's illness because cellular therapies are not usually believed effective against advanced cancers.

Kuhnau gives patients umbilical-cord cells and also thymus extract, the latter derived from a gland directly involved in antibody production. Hypothalamus, limbic, and brain-stem cells are also used because of their alleged influence on immunity and hormonal activity. Kuhnau and other alternative physicians also use live cells from shark tissues. Recent research has linked shark cartilage with tumor inhibition (sharks rarely develop cancer even when exposed to dangerous carcinogens). Several studies have also shown that shark tissues can constrict blood vessels which feed malignant tumors.[10]

Dr. Kuhnau cautions that an improper choice of live cells by inexperienced clinicians can lead to treatment failures. He cites a hypothetical example in which a patient suffers from thyroid and adrenal gland deficiencies. While some physicians might administer thyroid and adrenal cells, Kuhnau argues that pituitary extract is the right choice—because the pituitary is the master gland that regulates thyroid and adrenal activity in the first place.[11] Kuhnau thus underscores the necessity of balancing live cell treatments to effect maximum results. He also warns against the use of anything but living cells, since other versions (powdered or "lyophilized" preparations, for instance) lack the "vital force" needed for healing.

The Cost of Therapy

Costs are variable depending on duration of treatment and number of injections. At American Biologics Medical Center in Mexico, for example, five days of live cell therapy costs $2,700 including hotel accommodations. Each injection is listed at $200.

Potential Dangers Associated With Therapy

Allergic reactions, anaphylactic shock, and death have been blamed on live cell injections.[12] Nerve inflammation and encephalitis are other reported side effects. Due to these serious reactions, German officials imposed a ban on whole-cell products (which are freeze-dried) but not live cell preparations. The ban was enacted in 1987.

Dr. Kuhnau emphatically disputes the dangers of properly administered live cells. Kuhnau explains that he has treated 40,000 patients during a forty-two-year medical career and has never once seen a severe or fatal reaction. Kuhnau blames the European deaths on abuse and overuse of treatment. According to the physician, only 2 or 3 live-cell injections consisting of no more than 6 different types of cells should be given to patients during a course of treatment. Treatments should also be spaced at six-month intervals. But German doctors were allegedly administering 40 to 50 different cells at one time.[13]

Although orthodox medicine refutes the premise of live cell therapy, provocative reports have surfaced among mainstream researchers. For example, the American press recently reported that Dr. Madrazo Navarro, a Mexican surgeon, achieved remarkable results when he grafted adrenal gland cells into areas of the brain associated with Parkinson's disease. The grafted cells apparently caused a regeneration of diseased brain tissues.

This report, along with other favorable ones published during the last several decades, does not validate the use of live cell treatment for cancer. However, since foreign cells have been shown to bind with and possibly regenerate host tissues, their potential for stimulating organs involved in tumor suppression warrants closer scrutiny.

Many "remissions" and "cures" have been reported from live cell therapy, although the majority of these have not been verified in double-blind, clinical trials. Therefore, the merits of each report should be weighed on a case-by-case basis and, whenever possible, corroborated via medical documentation.

Improper manufacturing and sterilization procedures may be linked to recent treatment-related health problems; while live cell proponents argue that dangerous side effects have resulted from overuse, evidence of viral contamination has surfaced. In one case, a woman died two weeks after receiving live cell injections made from brain tissues. Investigators later found that viruses grew in the tissues.[14]

Those considering live cell therapy are thus urged to consult only well-established clinics with extensive experience. Whenever possible, patient records should be carefully reviewed and any treatment related problems assessed.

For further information contact

Sierra Clinic Inc.
30003 Gobernador Logo, Suite 202
Tijuana, Mexico
011 52-66-864672

Wolfram Kuhnau, M.D.
American Biologics
1180 Walnut Avenue
Chula Vista, CA 91911
1 (619) 429-8200
1 (800) 227-4458
1 (800) 227-4473

Program for Studies of Alternative Medicine
Hector E. Solorzan, M.D., Ph.D.
Universidad de Guadalajara
Calle Escuela Militar de Aviacion #16
Sector Hidalgo
Guadalajara, Jal.
Mexico
36-166155
36-157395
36-301094

DMSO

Dimethyl sulfoxide (abbreviated DMSO) was first used in the paper industry as a solvent. Medically, it is alleged to possess a broad spectrum of benefits against pain, arthritis, cancer, and other diseases.

Several studies have shown that DMSO can influence favorable conditions in the body by "scavenging" dangerous free radicals; free radicals are known to damage healthy cells and have been linked with cancer.

Since DMSO can readily pass through skin and other bodily membranes, some doctors use it to shuttle other medications into desired organs and tissues. DMSO is thus used concomitantly with cancer drugs or other substances such as vitamin C and Laetrile to assist in the absorption of those agents.

Studies Conducted on DMSO in Cancer Treatment

Several experiments in the 1960s claimed to substantiate DMSO's positive use in cancer therapy. For example, scientists working at Roswell Park Memorial Institute in Buffalo, New York, said that DMSO helped aid in the destruction of tumor metastases (i.e., spreading cells).[1] In another study, when DMSO was combined with a type of dye, it was found to kill malignant cells.[2]

According to Mrs. Mildred Miller, president of the Degenerative Disease Medical Center in Las Vegas, DMSO when used as part of a "metabolic" treatment regimen (including vitamins, Laetrile, enzymes and detoxifying enemas), can effect cancer remissions and even cures. She bases this claim on a study involving thirty brain cancer patients who, after DMSO treatment, reportedly experienced various degrees of remission. This study, however, has not been published in the peer-review literature.[3]

Why DMSO is Disputed

The American Cancer Society (ACS) says that a 1981 search of the medical and scientific literature revealed no "evidence" of anticancer benefit from DMSO. Oddly, the ACS reported that this conclusion was reached by "two consultants" (similar to the description of "two consultants" given in the ACS review of Iscador, chapter 12).

The National Academy of Sciences also stated that its 1982 review of all the pertinent literature did not justify approval of DMSO as a cancer drug.[4] Finally, researchers in a 1988 study combined DMSO with other drugs for the treatment of bladder cancer and found no increase in the absorption of the drugs. Interestingly, the manufacturer of a federally approved DMSO drug (not used in cancer treatment) stated that dimethyl sulfoxide does, in fact, potentiate (i.e., increase) the effectiveness of other concomitantly administered medications.[5] Exactly what these "medications" are, however, is not specified.

In any case, a number of independent studies performed *after* 1988 appear to contradict the ACS's negative assessment on DMSO. For example, one team of researchers found that DMSO could increase the cell-killing potential of cancer drugs.[6] In another report published in 1993, Swiss researchers discovered that DMSO incurred a significant survival advantage among patients suffering from advanced colon cancer.[7] In addition, other favorable reports have recently appeared in the peer-review literature.

The Only Currently Accepted Use of DMSO in the United States

Dimethyl sulfoxide has only been approved for use in the treatment of urinary bladder inflammation and is designated by the brand name "Rimso-50." Typically, a 50-milliliter dose of the drug (approximately 17 fluid ounces) is delivered directly into the bladder via a catheter. This treatment is repeated every few weeks until the inflammation subsides.

According to Rimso-50's manufacturer, DMSO has not been "approved as being safe and effective for any other" medical condition.[8]

Current research suggests that DMSO may have potential use as an adjunct in cancer chemotherapy. While further investigation is clearly warranted, holistic clinics use the drug in combination with a number of different treatments, including Laetrile and vitamin C.

DMSO is a relatively safe drug, but eye problems have occurred in several animal studies. For example, monkeys, dogs, and rabbits given high doses of DMSO developed physical changes in their lenses (i.e., the transparent structure behind the pupils). Lens changes can lead to conditions such as cataracts, in which vision is impaired. There is no evidence, however, that therapeutic doses of DMSO given under controlled conditions will cause eye problems. In any case, physicians recommend full eye evaluations for persons using the drug.

Anyone considering DMSO as an adjunctive cancer treatment should do so under careful supervision and in an experienced, clinical setting.

For further information contact:

Manufacturer of RIMSO-50:
Research Industries Corporation
Pharmaceutical Division
1847 West 2300 South
Salt Lake City, UT 84119

DMSO Therapy in Cancer:
Michael B. Schachter, M.D., P.C.
Two Executive Blvd.
Suffern, NY 10901
(914) 368-4700

FIFTEEN

Macrobiotics

Macrobiotics, originally called the "zen microbiotic diet," was first developed by the philosopher George Ohsawa in the 1950s. Ohsawa theorized that cancer and other diseases result from an imbalance in the two opposing yet interconnected forces of the universe known as "yin" and "yang." Popular to Oriental philosophy, yin and yang represent feminine and masculine, respectively. According to this philosophy, yin is a constantly expanding force and yang, a contracting one. In order for nature to exist in a state of harmony, yin and yang must exist in a state of balance. Consequently, an excess of one may lead to a deficiency in the other.

In the macrobiotic theory of cancer, a departure from the natural laws governing diet can affect the yin and yang balance, which is crucial to health. This can then result in a "toxic" condition ultimately leading to cancer.

While Ohsawa was the earliest proponent of macrobiotics, the system as it is currently practiced owes much of its popularity to Michio Kushi, a Japanese native. Kushi, who received degrees in political science and international law from Tokyo University, immigrated to the United States in the early 1960s. He later established the Kushi Institute in Massachusetts and became the internationally recognized leader of the macrobiotic health movement.

Macrobiotic Theory of Cancer Development

Macrobioticists point to a number of dietary factors. For example, overconsumption—or as Kushi calls it, "overnutrition"—of inappropriate foods can lead to a toxic condition in the body, resulting in cancer. Kushi also believes that "extreme" foods high in acid (meat, eggs, poultry, dairy products, fats, oils, and refined foods) derange the body's metabolism and provoke abnormal cell growth.[1] One example of this derangement occurs when overconsumption of acidic foods leads to a greater production of mucous in such organs as the lungs; according to Kushi, "fatty" deposits may then form which eventually result in cellular abberations that lead to cancer.

For this reason, Kushi urges that people eat more alkaline (or nonacidic) foods, including vegetables, cereals, and grains.

The Macrobiotic Diet

In general, the diet consists of 50 to 60 percent whole cereal grains, 5 percent soups, 25 to 30 percent vegetables, 5 to 10 percent beans and sea vegetables (kombu, wakame, nori, dulse), and, occasionally, seafood, fruits, nuts, and seeds.[2] After macrobiotic counselors diagnose patients' "yin/yang" requirements, they modify and customize the diet to suit individual needs.

The exotic nature of the diet with its avoidance of most traditional Western fare and its emphasis on specific cooking practices (electricity is prohibited; pressure cooking, steaming, and boiling are allowed) demands tremendous dedication by the dieter. In fact, macrobiotic proponents recommend that patients' families also follow the macrobiotic lifestyle, or, if this is not possible, that patients join a macrobiotic center or community for dietetic support and counseling.

Research on the Effectiveness of Macrobiotic Foods Against Cancer

Macrobiotic foods have been shown to prevent tumor incidence and block tumor growth.

In one study, miso soup—one of the common staples of the macrobiotic diet—was found to reduce the incidence of stomach cancer, 33 percent.[3] In another study conducted at the Harvard School of Public Health, rats that were fed kombu developed far fewer mammary cancers than rats not eating the plant. Moreover, kombu was found to show "consistent antitumor activity."[4] Other studies also corroborate the anticancer properties of seaweed.[5]

A further link between macrobiotics and cancer prevention is believed to exist because the diet contains a number of foods rich in vitamins, minerals, and other substances known to inhibit tumors. For example, leafy green and orange and yellow vegetables (kale, collard greens, spinach, squash, carrots) contain generous amounts of vitamins A and C as well as beta-carotene; these nutrients can all prevent cancer formation. In addition, cruciferous vegetables (cabbage, broccoli, Brussels sprouts, kohlrabi) contain a potent chemical known as *indole glycosinate* which has been found to protect against cancer.

Several studies have also shown that macrobiotics can extend the life span of advanced cancer patients.

One highly impressive trial was conducted by Dr. Vivian Newbold, a Philadelphia physician. In 1983, Dr. Newbold's husband was diagnosed with terminal, medically incurable colon cancer and he was given six months to live. After a period of macrobiotic treatment, Mr. Newbold went into remission. Eight months after his diagnosis, follow-up CAT scans showed 70 percent of the cancer was gone.[6]

When attempts to stimulate interest in her husband's unusual remission failed, Dr. Newbold implemented a small trial at her "own expense." The study consisted of six people with "medically incurable" cancers, including those of the pancreas, colon, liver, and abdomen.

After several years of follow-up, Newbold reported that four of her six patients experienced significant or total remission. In one case, a patient with incurable pancreatic cancer was alive and well nine years after diagnosis; in another, malignant melanoma remained in complete remission for nine years.

The two patients who did not respond went off their diet or made allowances that are forbidden (for example, switching from gas to electric cooking).[7]

Some critics suggest that the highly unusual remissions reported by Dr. Newbold may have resulted from conventional therapies initially received by her patients or from "spontaneous remissions."

Dr. Newbold argues that all currently used therapies are considered only palliative against the types of severe cancers afflicting her patients. Further, spontaneous remissions are so rare that their multiple occurrence in one small study group defies statistical probability, according to the physician.[8] In any case, the Newbold study, though highly impressive is not considered "proof" of efficacy simply because of its limited size.

In another study conducted by researchers at the Tulane School of Public Health, twenty-four macrobiotically treated patients with confirmed cancers of the pancreas were compared with matched controls.

After following their patients for over a year, the researchers reported a dramatic finding. The macrobiotic patients' average length of survival was 17.3 months, compared with only 6 months for the controls; remarkably, 54.2 percent of the macrobiotic patients were alive after one year against only 10 percent of the untreated control patients.[9] Although the researchers admitted that these results "were statistically significant" they claimed that other factors may have accounted for the superior macrobiotic responses, including a positive mental attitude.[10]

The American Cancer Society Position on Macrobiotics

The ACS disputes macrobiotics as a cancer therapy, arguing that positive treatment reports are based on personal testimonials and contain little scientific basis.[11] One such testimonial involved the story of Dr. Anthony Sattilaro, a physician who claimed a complete macrobiotically induced remission for his own incurable prostate cancer. Sattilaro's story attracted national attention and he wrote a best-selling book about his "cure."[12] But the ACS points out that the physician eventually died from his cancer.[13] (Interestingly, the ACS does not mention Dr. Newbold's study or the Tulane findings in its critique.)

The ACS also warns that, because macrobiotic diets are low in fat and simple sugars, they may cause problems in cancer patients experiencing weight loss and requiring increased amounts of protein and starch.[14] In addition, such diets may not be adequate for growing children whose nutritional needs are high, according the agency.

Based on these considerations, the ACS recommends that cancer patients eat foods high in animal protein to compensate for caloric abnormalities. But macrobioticists cite examples of patients who suddenly relapsed after being advised to add milk, meat, poultry, and other "forbidden" foods to their diet.[15]

Adverse Effects Associated with Macrobiotics

According to one report, a number of people practicing macrobiotics developed vitamin B-12 deficiencies.[16] In another report, 300 Dutch children on the diet developed rickets—a rarely seen disease caused by the lack of vitamin D. In addition, the growth curves of the children were below normal.[17]

Other reports contradict these findings. Canadian researchers found, for example, that people following a strict macrobiotic regimen did not suffer from any nutrient deficiencies and had normal vitamin and calcium levels in their blood. The researchers also discovered their subjects to have "superior" blood cholesterol levels.[18]

Some research has shown that a macrobiotic diet can inhibit and prevent tumor growth. In a few human trials, remarkable results were noted for otherwise incurable cancers. These trials have been criticized for a number of reasons, but pending data to the contrary, they still offer some corroboration for the disputed role of diet in cancer treatment.

Advocates of the macrobiotic diet say that it is generally safe and nutritious and meets established dietary guidelines. But the ACS considers the diet's limitations on animal protein, dairy products, and starches a cause for concern. Actually, both views might be correct. For example, people who have higher nutritional requirements (i.e., growing children or adults under the stress of chemotherapy or surgery) may indeed experience nutritional deficiencies on a macrobiotic program whereas healthy individuals might not.

Cancer patients using macrobiotics should thus consider periodic vitamin and mineral evaluations (many nutritionists and orthomolecular physicians routinely perform such tests). In many cases, daily supplementation with a B-12 tablet is all that will be needed to prevent complications; in other cases, a more aggressive vitamin program may be required. Check with your doctor.

Although some macrobioticists argue that vitamins can cause "chaos" in the body, Michio Kushi admits that supplementation has its place and is occasionally necessary.[19]

Those seeking macrobiotic treatment should only do so under the supervision of a trained counselor. Close collaboration with a holistic physician sympathetic to this form of therapy is also an option to consider.

For further information contact:

Kushi Institute of the Berkshires
P.O. Box 7
Becket, MA 01223
(413) 623-5741

Los Angeles East West Center
11215 Hannum Avenue
Culver City, CA 90230
(310) 398-2228

SIXTEEN

Vitamins, Minerals, and Enzyme Preparations in Cancer Treatment

While there has been much controversy and discussion over the use of vitamins to treat cancer and AIDS, a number of alternative physicians routinely use nutrients in cancer treatment. These substances are often given in megadoses hundreds or thousands of times greater than the recommended daily allowances.

Nutrient therapies are generally used in two ways. Some physicians and clinics incorporate them in an overall metabolic program—as discussed in chapter 17. Others use specific nutrients as a primary treatment. Depending on the physician, modalities such as chemotherapy and radiation are sometimes combined with nutrient therapies.

Nutrients Commonly Used in Cancer Therapy

Vitamins A, C, and E are believed to possess the most anticancer activity. The minerals selenium, germanium, molybdenum, tellurium, magnesium, and zinc are also being considered for their possible treatment value; of these minerals, scientists have been paying the most attention to selenium.

Enzymes are also used in alternative cancer treatment. Some clinicians administer enzymes intravenously to "dissolve" tumors.

Metabolic physicians credit these preparations with causing rapid and dramatic "liquidation" of tumor tissues.

Some Benefits of Vitamin A

A significant body of research shows vitamin A to play a crucial role in cancer prevention; there is little disagreement over the vitamin's preventive value.[1] Studies have also shown vitamin A's potential in cancer treatment.

One team of investigators found that vitamin A could reverse the growth of environmentally induced stomach and cervical cancers in animals.[2] Scientists also discovered that vitamin A enhanced the therapeutic effect of cancer drugs.[3] Beta carotene, which is chemically related to vitamin A, has also been found to prevent and even neutralize cancers, including those afflicting the lungs.*[4]

Orthodox researchers have also shown an interest in synthetically manufactured versions of vitamin A to treat cancer. Although similar to over-the-counter vitamins, these preparations are marketed through the pharmaceutical industry and can only be prescribed by a physician. One such medication is Accutane, which has been generally used to treat acne. In recent studies, the drug was found to prevent recurrences of head, neck, and skin malignancies

Pending further study, the American Cancer Society (ACS) has not yet endorsed regular vitamin A supplementation in cancer treatment.

Benefits Claimed by Holistic Cancer Physicians for Vitamin A

One of the world's leading advocates of vitamin A in cancer treatment is Robert Janker, founder of the Janker clinic in Bonn, Germany. Dr. Janker gives patients an emulsified version of vitamin A in order to reduce liver toxicity. Using this emulsion, Janker has been able to treat cancer patients with doses as high as *1.5 million units* daily. (This massive amount is 300 times greater than the recommended vitamin A allowance of 5,000 units per day). In addition to vitamin A, Janker and his colleagues use enzymes, immunity-boosting vaccines, and traditional therapies.

---

*Despite these and other positive reports which have appeared for over half a century, the National Cancer Institute has only recently begun to study vitamin A and its related substances known as retinoids and carotenoids in the prevention and treatment of cancer.

According to noted science writer Patrick McGrady, Janker has successfully treated over 50,000 seriously ill cancer patients for a 70 percent remission rate. The German physician has gone on record proclaiming that his multicombinational treatment doubles the life span of lung cancer patients (compared to patients receiving only radiation therapy) and causes some cancers of the reproductive organs to regress completely.

Other physicians have also claimed success with vitamin A. Among these were Dr. Max Gerson, who administered high amounts of the vitamin in the form of raw-pressed vegetable juices (see chapter 2), and Virginia Livingston, who gave her patients large amounts of juices and fruits high in abscisic acid—a vitamin A analog said to possess tumor-inhibiting qualities (see chapter 3).

How Minerals Are Used in Cancer Treatment

Selenium, a trace mineral with antioxidant properties, is considered one of the most powerful anticancer minerals known. While selenium's use in cancer treatment is still being investigated, it has shown powerful preventive effects. In one study, for example, selenium protected animals from developing cancers of the colon, liver, breast, and skin.[5] In another animal study, selenium reduced tumor incidence by nearly half—but only when combined with vitamin E.[6]

In the treatment of cancer, selenium is sometimes given in potentially toxic doses (a normal daily range is between 50 and 200 micrograms). A "non-toxic" version is also administered in doses normally considered dangerous.

One of the first physicians to claim success with high-dose selenium treatment was the highly controversial Emanuel Revici. Despite years of squabbling with medical review boards, Revici's concepts on selenium (and other aspects of cancer treatment) have been independently substantiated.[7]

In addition to selenium, scientists are also investigating the potent anticancer mineral germanium.

Japanese scientists were the first to synthesize an organic form of germanium (calling it "Ge-132") and to study the mineral's effects against various forms of cancer. Experiments have shown that Ge-132 can extend the life span of animals with cancer[8] and also slow down the development of lung cancer in mice.[9] Germanium also increases the production of tumor-killing interferons and antibodies.

Only the organic form of germanium is safe when taken in properly supervised doses; other forms, such as germanium oxide, are linked to kidney damage.

Enzymes Against Cancer

Enzymes were first proposed as a cancer treatment by Professor John Beard, a Scottish embryologist.

In 1902, Beard published a controversial thesis on the causation of cancer. According to Beard, cancer results when displaced cells in the body (known as "trophoblasts") are stimulated by estrogen and begin reproducing wildly. Beard believed that enzymes secreted by the pancreas could destroy these cells. He then administered pancreas enzymes to cancer patients, but this treatment did not work. However, later observers felt that Beard's enzymes were not correctly prepared or of proper strength.

Since Beard's initial experiments, enzyme technology has advanced substantially; a number of holistic doctors now claim success with enzyme combinations in the treatment of cancer.

Research on Enzymes and Cancer

In the 1960s, Dr. Frank Shively, a surgeon affiliated with the Ohio State Medical Association, treated his patients with a combination of five *proteolytic* (i.e., protein-digesting) enzymes. Shively claimed that intravenous and oral administration of his preparation literally caused tumors to liquefy and dissolve. The physician also reported numerous remissions involving over 100 bona fide cases of cancer.[10]

German scientists also experimented with newer enzyme formulations and proclaimed even better results. A pioneer in this research was Dr. Karl Ransberger who helped develop a formulation called "Wobe-Mugos." Wobe-Mugos contains enzymes from pancreas, calf thymus, papaya, and other sources, and when injected directly into tumors, is believed to weaken the outer tissues of cancer cells, leaving them susceptible to attack by the immune system.

After extensive use, Dr. Ransberger and Dr. Janker reported that a combination of Wobe-Mugos and vitamin A effected remissions in a number of cancer patients.[11] Other researchers noted similar effects, including a lowered recurrence of tumor growth[12] and a reduction in tumor mass.[13]

While enzyme therapy is not approved or endorsed by the American Cancer Society, positive laboratory experiments by orthodox researchers have taken place. One intriguing study involved a virus-derived enzyme known as *neuraminidase*. When scientists exposed cancer cells to this enzyme, protective growth hormone molecules on the cells were neutralized, leaving tumors more vulnerable to the immune system (see also chapter 3). This experiment was later published in the *Journal of the National Cancer Institute*.[14]

For years, health advocates cited the importance of daily nutrient supplementation, but they often encountered skepticism and even ridicule from the scientific community. Eventually, scientists—unable to deny the accumulation of hundreds of positive studies—accepted the validity of these claims. And while a good deal of skepticism still remains over the use of nutrients in cancer treatment, mainstream researchers are now beginning to give this area consideration as well. In fact, the National Cancer Institute is now sponsoring over twenty studies on vitamins A, C, E, beta carotene, and selenium in both cancer treatment and prevention.

Although there is no indisputable evidence that vitamins and minerals can cure cancer, many cancer patients feel that a judicious use of nutrients cannot hurt and may favorably alter the course of their illness.

Those considering supplementation should bear in mind that real dangers exist. Beside the risks already noted for germanium and selenium, metallic elements such as iron and copper are also potentially toxic. The oil-soluble vitamins A and D can be dangerous and megadoses of vitamin B-6 are linked to nerve damage. (Note: This is not a full summary of *all* the nutrients that are toxic.)

It is highly recommended that individuals who plan to follow a nutrient program familiarize themselves with the many facets of supplementation; a number of published sources that can supply valuable information are listed in the appendix. Patients are also advised to seek the advice of an orthomolecular physician or clinician experienced in this form of therapy.

(Note: Because metabolic cancer clinics also offer individual nutrient therapies, some of the clinics listed below are also found in "Metabolic Cancer Therapy" chapter 17. For reader convenience, an "L" after the clinic title indicates that the clinic has been listed there.)
    For further information contact:

High-dose vitamin A combined with enzymes. Also, alternative and orthodox modalities:

Robert Janker Clinic
Wolfgang Scheef, M.D.
Fachklinik für Tumorerkrankungen
Baumschulallee 12-14
5300 Bonn 1, Germany
011 49-228-7291-0

High-dose vitamin A plus full metabolic program:

Manner Clinic (L)
P.O. Box 434290
San Ysidro, CA 92143-4290
1-800-248-8431
011-526-680-4422

High-dose vitamin A plus BCG, selenium, and orthodox therapies:

Richard P. Huemer, M.D.
406 Southeast 131st Avenue, C-303
Vancouver, Washington 98684
(800) 444-1696
(205) 253-4445

High-dose selenium plus other elements, lipids, other:

Institute of Applied Biology (Emanuel Revici, M.D.)
26 East 36th Street
New York, NY 10016
(212) 685-0111

Intravenous germanium plus wide-range metabolic program:

Michael B. Schachter, M.D.
Two Executive Boulevard, #202
Suffern, New York 10901
(914) 368-4700

Germanium therapy plus other nutrients, enzymes, herbs, oxygen treatments, diet:

Atkins Center for Complementary Medicine
152 East 55th Street
New York, NY 10022
(212) 758-2110

Enzymes plus wide-range metabolic program including psychological/sensory therapies:

American Biologics (L)
1180 Walnut Avenue
Chula Vista, CA 91911
(619) 429-8200
(800) 227-4473

Enzymes plus wide-range metabolic program and spiritual counseling:

Hospital Ernesto Contreras
Paseo de Tijuana #1

Playas de Tijuana, B.C. 22700
Mexico
011 526-680-1850
(800) 700-1850

Mantell Medical Clinic
6505 Mars Rd.
Evans City, PA 16033
(412) 776-5610

SEVENTEEN

Metabolic Cancer Therapy

A number of clinicians combine many of the treatments discussed throughout this book in an attempt to offer the best chances of combating cancer. This type of eclectic approach, known as metabolic cancer therapy, focuses on restoring healthy immune function and potentiating the body's "natural" cancer-fighting abilities.

The modalities commonly used in metabolic treatment include Laetrile, vegetarian diets, "detoxifying" enemas, vitamins, enzymes, and a combination of intravenous as well as oxygen therapies. Some clinics administer the "Manner cocktail" (named after the late biochemist Harold Manner) which consists of high-dose vitamin C, Laetrile, and the drug DMSO.

The American Cancer Society (ACS) does not approve of any metabolically oriented therapies and disagrees with the premise on which they are based.

Metabolic Therapies Tested in a Clinical Setting

Dr. Harold Manner was one of the first scientists to test a metabolic cancer approach in the laboratory. In 1977, Manner conducted a controversial experiment in which he administered Laetrile, enzymes, and vitamin A to mice with cancer. One week after treatment, Manner reported a 90 percent total regression of cancer in the mice.

The study was done at the height of the Laetrile controversy, and its positive outcome was seen by Laetrile advocates as a boon to their cause. Cancer experts immediately criticized the study, not because it was a failure but because Laetrile and the other treatments were not examined single-handedly, according to usual protocol.

In order to resolve this criticism, Manner launched a second study (see Figure 1). This time, 550 mice with breast cancer were divided into 10 groups. Different combinations of Laetrile and/or enzymes and/or vitamins were given to deduce which had the most effect. After thirty days, Manner found that whatever the combination used, enzymes had to be involved in order for any positive effects to occur. Manner also found that the mice receiving Laetrile and enzymes, as well as the group receiving vitamin A and enzymes showed no more benefit than the group of mice receiving enzymes alone. Significantly, the mice that responded best received the total combination of vitamins, enzymes, and Laetrile.[1]

Despite this study, Manner was criticized for promoting a "spurious style of science" and for endorsing unproven cancer treatments.[2]

While the ACS has officially repudiated Manner and considers his research negligible, ACS officials do admit that enzymes, which form an important part of metabolic treatment, can, in fact, dissolve malignant tissues "in much the same manner that meat is digested by meat tenderizer"[3] (see also chapter 16).

Figure 1
Study Assessing the Effectiveness of Combination Laetrile, Enzymes, and Vitamin A in Cancer Treatment

Treatment (based on 50 mice)	Number totally regressing	% of total
Laetrile, vitamin A, enzymes	38/50	76
Laetrile, enzymes	27/50	54
vitamin A/enzymes	26/50	52
enzymes alone	26/50	52
Laetrile, vitamin A	0/50	0
Laetrile alone	0/50	0
vitamin A alone	0/50	0

Dr. Manner's Credentials

The scientist received his doctoral degree from Northwestern University in 1952 and later served as assistant professor, associate professor, and professor of biology at Syracuse University. During the 1970s, Manner was appointed chairman of the biology department at Loyola University in Chicago. He also wrote a number of scientific papers and articles.

While at Loyola, Manner founded the Metabolic Research Foundation, located in Glenview, Illinois.

Types of Programs Offered by Metabolic Clinics

Most clinics use diets, vitamins, minerals, enzymes, and Laetrile as described throughout this book. But depending on the clinic, a wide range of other treatments may be prescribed. For example, American Biologics of Mexico uses a number of therapies that include hydrazine sulfate, vaccines, live cell injections, and electromedicine.[4]

American Metabolic Institute combines traditional metabolic therapy with detoxifying enemas made from cancer-resistant shark cartilage, a special diet tailored according to blood type (patients with type-O blood are allowed animal protein, while A and B blood types are given vegetable foods), hydrogen peroxide, homeopathy, ultrasound, and other strategies. The institute's director, Geronimo Rubio, M.D., also administers a variety of vaccines, which include *active*, *passive*, and *non-specific* types made from patients' tumor tissues and white blood cells. "Blocking proteins" (which appear to resemble Burton's Immuno-Augmentative method) are also employed.[5]

According to Dr. Rubio, fifteen patients who had been suffering from "incurable cancers of the lung, pancreas and breast" were still found to be in remission seven years after being treated with his method.[6]

A popular but highly controversial treatment also being used by some metabolic clinics is chelation therapy. Chelation (pronounced kē'lā shən) is approved for the treatment of lead and other metal poisonings but not for cancer. Chelating agents work by attracting metal ions (i.e., electrically charged atoms) and drawing them out of the body. The drug EDTA (ethylenediaminetetraacetic acid) is a common chelator that has proven useful for metal poisoning. After intravenous administration with the drug, unwanted ions are eliminated through the urine.

A number of alternative clinicians use chelation to "increase" blood circulation in their cancer patients, a factor they believe crucial to reversing the malignant process. This theory is based on the assumption that EDTA and other chelators improve blood flow by removing atherosclerotic plaques from the arteries.

Orthodox doctors strongly disagree with this claim, but some physicians believe that EDTA may offer a cheaper alternative to bypass surgery.

The ACS does not agree with nor accept the practice of metabolic cancer therapy. Not only are the individual treatments controversial, but standard scientific testing is generally geared toward assessing one therapy at a time. According to critics, it is impossible to tell which treatment is effecting what result in a metabolic program. Others point out, however, that multicombinational therapies can be tested by studying groups of people receiving different treatment combinations, as Dr. Manner did in his revised animal experiments.

In the absence of any rigorous scientific trials, one clue to possible benefits from metabolic therapy comes from a scientific inquiry of cancer patients so treated. When questioned, 64 percent of the patients claimed to have either been cured or greatly helped. In addition, 73 percent felt their general health to have improved.[7] Of course, these percentages are not seen as scientific proof of benefit but may help to gauge how cancer patients perceive and are affected by metabolic treatment.

Those considering a metabolic cancer program should examine each clinic's regimen carefully, including the individual therapies offered. The scientific references outlined in this book will serve as a helpful starting point for investigation.

Different clinics may claim better results for select types of cancer, so it is recommended that those seeking treatment check on this matter thoroughly. Speak with patients and review the medical records of many clinics.

NOTE: Because metabolic cancer clinics also offer individual nutrient therapies, some of the clinics listed below are also found in chapter 16 ("Vitamins, Minerals, and Enzyme Preparations in Cancer Treatment"). For the reader's convenience, an "L" after the clinic indicates that the clinic has already been listed.

For further information contact:

Manner Clinic (L)
P.O. Box 434290
San Ysidro, CA 92143-4290
1 (800) 248-8431
(526) 680-4422

American Biologics (L)
1180 Walnut Avenue
Chula Vista, CA 91911
(619) 429-8200
(800) 227-4473

American Metabolic Institute
524 Calle Primera Road, Suite 1005A
San Ysidro, CA 92173
(619) 229-3003
(800) 388-1083

EIGHTEEN

Adjuvant Vaccine Therapies

Cancer clinics that combine a wide range of unorthodox treatments—including vaccines—are considered "metabolic" or "alternative." A number of physicians, however, do not ascribe to the premise of alternative medicine but still offer vaccines designed to stimulate immunity and supplement traditional therapies. These physicians generally work within the framework of organized medicine, publish their data, and avoid criticizing established forms of medicine.

While adjuvant vaccine regimens (also called "immunotherapy") are often considered experimental and not a usual aspect of orthodox medicine, their use has become more tolerated by the mainstream. Part of that tolerance seems motivated by a public insistent on expanding its health care options.

Dr. Burton A. Waisbren, head of the Waisbren clinic in Milwaukee, Wisconsin, is a leading proponent of adjuvant vaccine therapy. Since the early 1970s, Dr. Waisbren has treated patients with Mixed Bacterial Vaccine, Bacillu, Calmette-Guérin (BCG), Transfer Factor, and Lymphoblastoid Lymphocytes.

Mixed Bacterial Vaccine (MBV) is made from the bacteria which infects burn patients and is believed to stimulate production of cancer-killing tumor necrosis factor. MBV has been safely administered to thousands of people with no apparent side effects.[1] Bacterial organisms that form the basis of Coley's toxins (see chapter 1) have also been used by Dr. Waisbren.

Transfer Factor (TF), which is made by taking special immune-system cells from healthy donors, is believed to help the body recognize and target cancer cells. The rationale for using Transfer Factor is based on earlier research which showed that breast cancer patients could respond favorably to this form of treatment.[2]

BCG, a common vaccine that has long been used to prevent tuberculosis, is believed to stimulate the pathogen-devouring activity of different immune-system cells. Made from strains of microorganisms known as *Mycoplasma*, BCG has been under investigation as an anticancer agent for over two decades.

Although BCG has been used for years, the serum's therapeutic potential in cancer treatment is only now being realized. Currently, BCG is widely used as an adjunctive therapy in bladder cancer.

Lymphoblastoid Lymphocytes are living white blood cells derived from various sources, including people under the stress of infection. These cells are believed to help the immune system reject cancer cells in the same way that donor organs are rejected by transplant recipients.[3]

Immunotherapy's Effectiveness Against Human Cancers

The type of immune-stimulating programs practiced by Dr. Waisbren and others are considered, at the very least, worthwhile adjuncts to standard therapies. In some instances, total or significant regression of tumors has occurred.

One woman suffering from Hodgkin's disease chose immunotherapy after toxic drugs caused a dangerous drop in her blood count. Cancerous nodes in the woman's neck and chest began to grow, and her condition deteriorated. After receiving a combination of vaccines, the woman's blood count returned to normal, her nodes "disappeared" and CAT, gallium, and bone scans were all negative for cancer.[4]

Another patient discontinued chemotherapy after doctors were unable to attain the toxic doses necessary to stop cancer growth in the lung and chest wall. Immunotherapy was started, and nearly ten years after diagnosis, CAT scans and X rays show no spread of cancer.[5] A number of other patients also showed positive responses to vaccine therapy.

In one study, for example, twenty-two lung cancer patients who received vaccines were compared with an untreated control group. Follow-up later showed that the vaccine patients lived, on average, nine months longer than their untreated counterparts.[6]

Immune-directed treatments were also shown to be effective against melanoma, lymphoma, leukemia, and cancers of the colon and breast.

Benefits of Immunotherapy

Dr. Waisbren feels that because of its relative safety, immunotherapy (and particularly BCG vaccine) should be used by all cancer patients.[7] According to Waisbren, such a program would offer the added insurance of increasing patients survival odds. For example, a woman who has a 75 percent probability of fully recovering from breast cancer might minimize the remaining 25 percent chance of relapse via immunotherapy.

In the case of a lung cancer patient whose odds of cure are only 20 percent, immunotherapy may offer an *only* chance at decreasing the dismal 80 percent likelihood of cancer recurrence.

In certain instances, vaccine strategies are used without any other treatment; this is likely to occur when patients' blood-forming systems are so weak that toxic therapies are ruled out, or when patients simply refuse standard treatment.

Treatment programs such as those practiced at the Waisbren clinic can cost between $3,000 and $8,000 per year.

The American Cancer Society's Position on the Use of Vaccines in Cancer Treatment

While a number of alternative vaccine strategies are showing promise, the ACS has not actively endorsed their use in cancer treatment.* However, the Food and Drug Administration has recently granted approval for the use of BCG in the treatment of bladder cancer.

Currently, most physicians have the legal right to dispense nonex-

---

*The ACS did remove Coley's toxins (a type of mixed bacterial vaccine) from its *Unproven Therapies List* recently, after new evidence corroborated the treatment's usefulness. Nonetheless, Coley's toxins and Mixed Bacterial Vaccine are still not being used in traditional cancer treatment.

perimental vaccines in the interest of their patients, as long as the vaccines are not sold for profit or commercial enterprise.

Many scientists consider adjuvant vaccine therapies a worthwhile approach in the treatment and possible prevention of cancer. In fact, a number of established research centers have begun clinical trials to test these immune-oriented strategies.

Unquestionably, a perceptible shift has occurred toward cancer treatments that are less tumor-targeted and more immunity-enhancing. Indeed, a small but growing number of physicians, disgruntled with the poor prognoses offered by toxic therapies, use adjuvant vaccines in the hope that survival odds will improve. But many orthodox practitioners are still reluctant to accept vaccine treatments that are "user friendly" and less expensive than those being pioneered by many biotechnological pharmaceutical concerns.

In fact, many of the immunological strategies under investigation (with the exception of BCG) appear to follow the same conceptual design as toxic cancer drugs. A case in point involves the much-touted Interleukin-2 (IL-2) under investigation at the National Institutes of Health; although some successes have been reported, IL-2 was found to provoke such serious side effects that its use has been curtailed and initial excitement over the drug has dampened. Conversely, the treatments outlined in this chapter cause a few side effects, which are usually mild and transient.

While the effectiveness of adjuvant vaccine therapies is still being debated, preliminary data show that they may indeed prove useful for those patients determined to lessen the odds of cancer recurrence. At this time, lymphomas and lung malignancies appear to be among the best responders to this form of therapy.

Before deciding on any vaccine program, check with the clinic, its protocol, and the type of cancers that have shown the best response.

For further information contact:

Waisbren Clinic
2315 North Lake Drive, Suite 815,
Seton Tower
Milwaukee, WI 53211
(414) 272-1929

NINETEEN

What You Need to Know
About Choosing an
Alternative Cancer Therapy

Of all the challenges facing cancer patients, one of the most formidable involves choice of therapy.

Countless questions plague patients and their families, but probably the most tortuous involves the decision to choose an alternative therapy. When should one make this difficult choice? What if abandoning conventionality puts the patient at greater risk? How efficacious is the considered alternative? How does one make a commitment to an "unproven" treatment in the face of inevitable criticism and isolation from the medical mainstream and sometimes even one's own family?

These and other questions present a serious dilemma, because the answers to them are usually made alone and without the support of one's attending physician or the endorsement of orthodox agencies such as the American Cancer Society (ACS) and National Cancer Institute (NCI). In spite of these difficulties, Americans have become increasingly active in mapping their own health care destinies.

The decision to adopt an active role in one's own health care can, in itself, be a key factor in promoting survival and well-being; Bernice

Wallen described this phenomenon in her book *I Beat Cancer*.[1] After conducting intensive research, Wallen decided that an unapproved course of treatment would offer the best hope for her incurable cancer. Literally dozens of physicians dissuaded the housewife, arguing that the type of vaccine treatment she had decided on would not prove beneficial. But Wallen persisted and then finally, after being accepted in a clinical trial, experienced a remarkable remission.

In addition to the question of choosing a therapy, other concerns are *when* and *how* it should be done. When making this difficult decision, you need to take a number of factors into consideration.

Choosing an Alternative Cancer Therapy

There is no consensus as to when an alternative treatment should be considered. But a set of guidelines that might be helpful were suggested by New York orthomolecular physician H. L. Newbold.

In his book *Vitamin C Against Cancer*, Newbold recommends that any tumor which can be surgically removed should be.* Many alternative practitioners agree, on the assumption that nontoxic, immune-stimulating therapies work better if there if less cancer in the body. Of course, some patients might refuse surgery if the disability and/or disfigurement do not appreciably affect survivability. But the decision to not undergo surgery can be complex and should never be made until all the data has been carefully assessed and discussed with health care professionals who are objective and open-minded.

Regarding toxic chemotherapy, Newbold describes an "odds" of survival factor. Accordingly, the decision to accept drug therapy is a respectable one when the odds for five-year survival** are in the 50 percent range.[2] Once the odds drop below 50 percent, the value of chemotherapy as a viable option diminishes proportionately. Newbold cites the example of a woman who, diagnosed with a particularly virulent form of cancer, is given a 30 percent five-year survival rate provided she takes the drug cis-platinum. But the woman's treatment will exact a heavy toll in terms of duration and side effects. Newbold argues that in this case, "the prospect of being deathly sick [from

---

*Newbold mentions several exceptions, including treatment-related disfigurement or impotence that may worsen the quality of life.

**The time frame which, in the absence of disease recurrence, constitutes a "cure" according to the American Cancer Society.

treatment]...." would not be very worthwhile based on the poor odds.[3]

In such cancers as those of the liver, esophagus, and pancreas, survival values plummet far below 50 percent. Still, some physicians might recommend vigorous treatment if for no other reason than to offer patients "hope." Others might advise against treatment, and a few physicians might be open to alternatives.

Even when conventional treatments are decided upon, people can and do supplement such programs. In Newbold's practice, cancer patients sometimes receive high doses of vitamin C to help fight their disease and to reduce toxic side effects from the drugs they may be receiving. Some physicians use other strategies in conjunction with standard treatments.

Many orthodox physicians will voice their opposition to supplementation with alternative therapies—often with great conviction. In this situation, one must consider whether the doctor's reaction is valid or biased. For example, a chemotherapist opposed to the use of hydrazine sulfate in a patient might cite hydrazine's "toxicity" or "unproven" efficacy. However, hydrazine has been proven far less toxic than any known cancer drug today, and efficacy has been established in a number of scientific studies (see chapter 4). In a case like this, it would be worthwhile to show the therapist corroborating studies along with all the available references.

To be sure, many informed and educated patients who are given relatively good odds choose not to undergo chemotherapy or radiation, in the belief that such treatments will adversely effect immunity and overall survival. Dr. Burton Waisbren, who has had long-term experience treating cancer, cites the fact that a large number of people "cannot or will not" accept chemotherapy or radiation.[4]

Of course, great care must be exercised when the decision not to embark on a "proven" course is made. Crucial to this decision lies the issue of a treatment's known benefits. For example, while some antileukemia drugs have proven themselves remarkably effective, other drugs used against certain types of lung cancer are considered only palliative and not curative. A distinction should thus be made based on a careful review of the known cure probabilities (cited throughout this book and elsewhere). In this matter, frank and open discussion with one's personal physician is always prudent, but if such dialogue is not fruitful, choosing another physician might be advisable.

When assessing a therapy, care must also be applied to the definition of "cure." Does cure mean a very good chance for five-year survival? Or does it suggest the possibility of remission followed by a debilitating life-style with no hopeful, long-term outcome? Unfortunately, the word "cure" can be ambiguous and open to interpretation. For example, the ACS considers Hodgkin's disease, acute myeloid leukemia, and ovarian cancer curable even in advanced stages.[5] However, by that agency's own data (as found in its annual report journal), acute myeloid leukemia has less than a 25 percent five-year survival ratio, and advanced ovarian cancer, an 18 percent cure rate.[6] That such cancers can, in fact, be successfully treated a small percentage of the time evidently connotes curability in the ACS's view. But from an odds standpoint, the outlook may be quite poor.

How to Choose an Alternative Therapy

Once a decision is made to augment a standard therapy regimen or to use an alternative method alone, a number of pointed questions must be addressed and resolved as best as possible. How effective is the desired treatment, and what types of cancers respond best? What are the cure or remission rates, and are there any medical records or clinical trials offering corroboration?

According to the ACS, the only proven and acceptable therapies are those that have been subjected to animal and human testing and whose results have been published in the peer-reviewed literature. All others that have not are immediately suspect. However, this assumption excludes many important factors—historical and otherwise. The fact is, not every alternative clinician can display published data, for a number of complex reasons; Lawrence Burton, who developed Immuno-Augmentative Therapy, was not able to find an interested publisher after his work started to generate controversy. Prior to that time, however, he was publishing scientific articles (see chapter 5). But even had Burton published extensively, it is questionable whether his controversial ideas would have found acceptance.

Consider that Virginia Livingston, the promoter of antibacterial cancer vaccines, *did* publish twelve peer-reviewed scientific papers but was still accused of never providing any data to support her theories (see chapter 3). Remarkably, Dr. Stanislaw Burzynski wrote nearly *one hundred* peer-reviewed papers and articles on his "antineoplaston" cancer therapy. Yet, antineoplastons have only recently begun gaining a modicum of acceptance, after years of rejection.

Other factors make published data hard to gather. For example, many people who travel to Mexico, Europe, and other countries for medical care do so in the late stages of cancer. Often the treatments they seek—while having the negative distinction of not being scientifically tested in humans—have not been adequately disproven either. In many cases, patients complete a therapy but do not maintain contact with the clinic. In other instances, patients die before any follow-up can be completed.

Another formidable problem is that many alternative clinics employ a variety of nontoxic modalities; this virtually guarantees nonacceptance from a medical mainstream intent on proving the value of single, *toxic* treatments for cancer. Due to this factor, Harold Manner's published study of cancer remission via a combination of Laetrile, vitamin A, and enzymes was negated (see chapter 17).

Whatever hardships alternative cancer clinics may indeed be facing, they are certainly not beyond scrutiny and should be questioned thoroughly before any agreement to be treated is made.

After contacting a clinic, do not hesitate to ask if you can see patients' medical records. While this is not always feasible because of privacy constraints, many clinics do keep some form of documentation on patients' case histories. Such information can serve as a good starting point for investigation.

Caution is urged when leafing through case reports. If, for instance, a patient is described as having had "cancer" which was diagnosed by a "local doctor" and after treatment, "appears" to be doing "well," there is reason for some skepticism; the cancer should have been exactly defined and the diagnosing doctor named. In addition, the phrase "appears to be doing well" is not a quantitative assessment and does not reveal anything; either the patient is or is not in remission, and verifiable tests and procedures should be listed which proclaim this in the history.

Here are other important questions you should ask when screening a clinic:

What are the physician's credentials? Not every alternative treatment center is run by a medical doctor, but this does not automatically negate the usefulness of a treatment. However, the clinician should have a degree in the sciences from an accredited university (and not, for example, a correspondence school).

What are the clinic's remission or cure percentages? While this may be difficult to verify, it can serve as a point of comparison when conducting separate interviews of patients. For example, if the clinic claims a 50 percent "cure" rate for lung cancer, but only 1 of the 5 lung-cancer patients interviewed has been cured, there is an obvious discrepancy.

When a clinic claims cures or remissions, what are they describing? Be careful of the distinction between "cure" and "remission." A patient claiming an improvement in symptoms for a span of only six months is not considered cured but may be in active remission. Also, be skeptical of any clinic that makes extravagant claims substantially different from known prognoses (for example, 80 percent cure rates for pancreas cancer which is usually 4 percent curable) without being able (or willing) to offer corroboration.

Does the clinic offer chemotherapy, radiation, and surgery? If not, are there affiliated hospitals that do? An alternative clinician that disputes *any* form of orthodox treatment without reviewing the individual circumstances should be considered suspect, because conventional therapies may be clearly warranted in some patients.

When documentation is available, it can help to put a clinic's sense of objectivity and honesty into perspective. For example, if a clinic states that "extensive data offers compelling proof for our treatment," but only one or two animal studies exists, further probing may be necessary to pin down just what "extensive data" means.

Valuable information that may also shed light on a clinic or treatment can be obtained through interviews with patients. After contacting a clinic, ask for and *expect* to speak with former patients; any clinic that advises against this screening process should be questioned. Telephone numbers can also be obtained from such organizations as the Cancer Control Society (see Appendix). Generally, people who are on telephone lists have volunteered to speak with others about their treatment experiences. Of course, this should never be assumed, so after contact is made, politely ask if the respondent is aware that their name was on a list and is willing to share information.

While the ACS categorically disputes the personal testimonial and considers it the least reliable source of information, many legitimate patient claims can be verified. It is important to remember, however, that a crucial difference exists between hearsay reports of benefit and bona fide cures.

According to the ACS, "cure" or "remission" testimonials can be misleading for the following reasons:

> Patients may have a form of cancer that is progressing slowly and not manifesting any symptoms but the alternative treatment is still credited with extending life span.

> Patients may have had a nonmalignant tumor that has essentially disappeared by itself but credit is given to the alternative treatment for curing the malignancy.

> Patients who have just recently received a course of standard therapy, then switched over to a holistic program, may be experiencing a regression due to the effects of the original treatment. But again, credit is given the alternative therapy.

An example of this last scenario occurred when a woman with early-stage breast cancer underwent surgery and a course of chemotherapy. The woman completely recovered but decided on the added "insurance" of a macrobiotic diet. In this case, the macrobiotic diet could not be said to have brought on the woman's recovery, although some might make such a claim.

In other cases, however, the unusual progress of a patient who begins an alternative therapy immediately after a course of standard treatment can serve as a useful barometer regarding the newly chosen treatment.

For example, one patient diagnosed with advanced lung cancer received an aggressive course of chemotherapy; this treatment was offered as a "last resort," but the patient's prognosis remained very poor. Then after embarking on a metabolic-vaccine regimen, the person experienced a verifiable remission that lasted several years. Although the ACS would probably cite the original therapy as a major factor in this remission, the odds were significantly against such a recovery. Therefore, *some* value may be applied to the alternative treatment.

Before assessing cure reports, it is important to verify that a person had cancer in the first place and if so, to what extent. Thus, the following questions should be satisfactorily answered:

Was the person's cancer identified via a biopsy?

Were specific tests and diagnostic procedures performed (for example, CAT scans, X rays, liver-function studies, etc.)?

Were these tests reviewed by a competent pathologist, radiologist, and physician in an accredited hospital or clinic?

It is also important to find out what *type* of malignancy the patient had. Usually, people who have been genuinely diagnosed and treated for cancer will be able to cite specific details. For example, a person who says "I was diagnosed with adenocarcinoma of the pancreas that spread to a node" is probably repeating, verbatim, an official medical report. A person saying "I had cancer all over the place" is not being specific and should be asked to provide further details.

Often, cure claims that occur outside the realm of established medicine—however legitimate they may be—will still be viewed with skepticism by the medical mainstream. One of the most common explanations offered by doctors is that the cure resulted from a "spontaneous remission"—i.e., the sudden, unexplained disappearance of a cancer not due to any known treatment or cause. Spontaneous remissions, however, are so rare that their alleged occurrence among alternative cancer patients defies any logical degree of probability.

According to an extensive study conducted by the Institute of Noetic Sciences in Washington, D.C., fewer than 1,000 documented cases of spontaneous remission in the world occurred between the years 1900 and 1987.[7] When one considers the total number of cancer deaths in that time frame (there were over *4 million* such deaths in the United

States alone during just the last *ten years*), the actual odds against a spontaneous remission occurring are hundreds of thousands of times to one. Nonetheless, spontaneous remissions are *routinely* used to account for unexplainable cures—especially when orthodox treatment methods have failed.

Buyer Beware

In the course of assessing all the information already described, it is also important to be on the lookout for signs of fraud or unethical behavior among health practitioners. While clinics who meet the basic criteria outlined here are more than likely legitimate, charlatans—in both alternative and mainstream medicine—do exist.

The ACS lists a number of keys that can signal deception, including the following:

The use of double-talk. Some unethical clinicians manipulate patients by using arcane or illogical phrases and terminologies. For example, the statement "your cancer can't be cured but you can" is a form of double-talk that has no known basis in either fact or common sense.

Weasel words. These are words or sentences used to promise prospective patients a great deal that, on closer inspection, actually guarantee nothing. For instance, the following advertisement was used to describe one company's alternative health product: "*Theoretically*, the nutrients found in this glandular supplement *may* contain essential factors that will *help* the body's glands." According to the ACS, the weasel words (italicized) actually promise nothing but superficially sound impressive.

Focusing on the positive. When a patient's condition is not improving, symptoms not yet materialized are used as a point of vindication. For example, if a patient has continuing pain in the right shoulder, it may be pointed out that the pain "hasn't gone into the left shoulder as expected" and this is a "positive" sign that a treatment is working. Such statements should be viewed very skeptically in the absence of proof to the contrary.

Questionable tests and other practices. While some of the tests employed by alternative practitioners may differ substantially from those used in mainstream medicine, their uniqueness does not automatically imply quackery. However, if broad and sweeping diagnoses or measurements of progress are made *solely* on the basis of such tests to the exclusion of all other standard protocols, one should be cautious. It may be that some therapists—such as macrobioticists who evaluate patients by *physiognomic* (i.e., visual) examination—are simply practicing metaphysical or ancient medical disciplines. Significantly, an alternative clinician's *openness* toward and utilization of established tenets of diagnosis can serve as an important measure of integrity.

Other Important Considerations

Once the decision is made to go ahead with an alternative therapy, patients must be prepared to stand by their convictions. Family physicians who are skeptical can be shown all the published citations quoted in this book and elsewhere regarding the treatment; when these are lacking, all pertinent data from patient interviews can be shared. Orthodox oncologists who are pressing for a vigorous course of chemotherapy—despite poor survival odds and the patient's belief that drugs will do more harm than good—can be asked to provide published studies corroborating the value of *their* treatments. Radiologists who are recommending therapy to shrink a fast-growing tumor can be asked to provide data on possible side effects, including the risks of acquiring secondary tumors.

When one's primary physician will not even consider an alternative approach nor be willing to review pertinent data, case histories or the results of treatment interviews, then it may be time to find another physician with a keen interest in holistic medicine.

Once a commitment is made, the patient should give a newly selected therapy a fair chance to work. In some cases, the treatment may last only several weeks; in others, such as the Gerson therapy, more than one year is the expected duration. It is therefore crucial that patients fully understand the time elements involved and that they be willing to plan their lives accordingly.

It is also important that patients have the strong support of family and friends to help them endure and cope with many of the obstacles they may imminently face. In fact, it is not uncommon for people to discontinue a treatment before completion because family members were not willing to adapt to the therapy's stringent guidelines. Significantly, patients *and* their families are advised to reach some common agreement concerning treatment choices and any difficulties liable to occur should be discussed and planned for ahead of time.

The following questions may help some families better determine how they collectively feel toward a selected therapy:

Does the family agree on the primary theory and philosophy of the therapy that is being considered?

Are patients and family comfortable that their review of all pertinent information has been satisfactory?

Have potential side effects, duration of treatment, and all other related variables been satisfactorily discussed?

Are family members willing to make the necessary modifications and adjustments to expedite therapy? For example, will the strict dietary guidelines of a Gerson or macrobiotic-type diet be adhered to or will social pressures create problems?

Will patients who are still working and traveling be able to faithfully continue their program (for example, by maintaining a food or vitamin regimen away from home)?

Are support groups a realistic option that family members would agree working with?

Disagreements over the above questions may jeopardize the commitment necessary to insure a treatment's potential success. Thus, frank and open discussion will help to lay bare any conflicts that might crop up at unexpected or disadvantageous times in the course of a patient's illness.

Finally, financial arrangements should be carefully discussed with the clinic of choice and the insurance company before commencing treatment. Many insurers will not cover the cost of alternative, experimental, or unproven cancer therapies, but many variables exist that may allow for some blanket coverage (for example, when an alternative clinic also offers a standard program not considered experimental). Be sure to have all covered costs spelled out ahead of time and preferably in writing.

TWENTY

Toward the Conquest of Cancer

W hile alternative cancer treatments have, in many cases, been reported to show highly favorable results, their use is still largely prohibited in the United States. Meanwhile, orthodox therapies which are said to cure only a minority of total cancer cases are heralded as the only truly effective treatments. Moreover, the industries that supply and design these treatments continue to enjoy billion-dollar profit margins, and this alone is cited by critics as a major factor in stalling acceptance of new, holistic ideas in cancer treatment.

Surely, certain gains have been made through the orthodox therapies and these rightly deserve acclaim. But the necessity of overhauling established dogma and its inherent opposition to competitive ideas and alternative strategies is being urged by many holistic-oriented clinicians who complain about the enormous cancer casualties *not* being ameliorated.

Ironically, Americans, who pride themselves as among the most advanced scientific cultures on earth and who view ancient medical practices with a degree of amusement and pity, may themselves bewilder and amuse future historians as a people who treated cancer by cutting, burning, and poisoning. And twentieth-century cancer medicine—despite all the hoopla about progress and high technology—may very well be looked at as having been worse than the disease itself.

Nonetheless, the philosophy and practice of conventional cancer medicine has been seriously challenged in the last decade. The alternative cancer movement, however history judges it, has forced a rethinking of long-held perceptions. Few people, whether scientist or citizen, would disagree that traditional concepts of treatment must be dramatically revised before the losing cancer war can finally be won.

Indeed, more Americans than ever before are choosing less toxic, naturally oriented treatments regardless of orthodoxy's admonitions not to do so. Public dissatisfaction with the failing "war on cancer" has also forced government officials to reappraise their own long-standing biases against the use of vitamins, herbs, diets, and other natural remedies long considered in the domain of quackery and charlatanism. In what has now become a new climate of openness, some alternative therapies once scoffed at and labeled as worthless are beginning to receive serious consideration. Such an affirmation would have been unthinkable two decades ago.

In 1990, the Office of Technology Assessment (OTA) completed a three-year evaluation on unconventional therapies at the urging of legislators and concerned citizens. This report did not vindicate the therapies but agreed that they deserved closer scrutiny. Although the report was criticized for being "closed-minded," physicians praised it for creating a "bridge" between the two "long-feuding" sides of the cancer issue. Following the OTA's report the National Institutes of Health (NIH) held its first workshop on Unconventional Medical Practices. The 1992 workshop was attended by physicians, scientists, and representatives of the Food and Drug Administration.

Participants discussed a wide variety of alternative treatments, including macrobiotics, metabolic therapies, homeopathy, herbal medicine, oxidation, cell therapies, and prayer, among many others. The workshop's attendees concluded that alternative therapies should receive more attention from the scientific community, less restraint from government agencies, and an outlet for peer review through scientific publications. In fact, the NIH already has in place an Office of Alternative Medicine.

Despite the unprecedented progress that has been made, a schism still exists between both sides of the cancer issue and this will undoubtedly continue for years to come. But an ever-increasing number of Americans are not waiting for the issue to be settled and have instead taken it upon themselves to investigate and utilize alternative treatments. Unfortunately, a disturbing lack of accurate and unbiased information exists on this complex subject—an ironic dilemma considering that most Americans regard the freedom to informed choice as an indisputable right.

Hopefully, the information in this book will help close the gap by offering people, in the quandary of decision making, scientifically valid and documented information on alternative cancer therapies, free from dogma, hysteria, and bias.

Appendix

Arlin J. Brown Information Center, Inc.,
P.O. Box 251
Fort Belvoir, VA 22060
(703) 752-9511

Cancer Control Society
2043 N. Berendo St.
Los Angeles, CA 90027
(213) 663-7801
(Books, tapes, patient/physician lists, bus tours to Mexican clinics, updates.)

Can Help
3111 Paradise Bay Rd.
Port Ludlow, WA 98365-9771
(206) 437-2291
(Information service customized to individual patients; offers current data and personalized packets for a fee.)

National Health Federation
212 West Foothill Blvd.
P.O. Box 688
Monrovia, CA 91016
(818) 357-2181
(Nonprofit organization dedicated to free choice in alternative medicine.)

Patient Rights Legal Action Fund
202 W. 78th Street, 3E
New York, NY 10024

(The organization that originally filed a suit on behalf of Dr. Stanislaw Burzynski.)

People Against Cancer
P.O. Box 10
Otho, Iowa 50569-0010
(515) 972-4444

World Research Foundation
15300 Ventura Blvd., Suite 405
Sherman Oaks, CA 91403
(818) 907-5483

(Disseminates published information on the medical literature past and present; an extensive data base can access medical articles and other materials pertinent to alternative cancer therapies.)

Project Cure
1101 Connecticut Avenue N.W.
Washington, D.C. 20036

American Association of Orthomolecular Medicine
7375 Kingsway
Burnaby, British Columbia, V3N 3B5 Canada

ORTHODOX CANCER/MEDICAL ORGANIZATIONS

American Medical Association
535 North Dearborn Street
Chicago, IL 60610
(312) 645-5000

National Cancer Institute
National Institutes of Health
Bethesda, MD 20892

American Cancer Society
1599 Clifton Rd., NE
Atlanta, GA 30329
(404) 320-3333
(800) ACS-2345

Notes

Preface

1. S. Louie and R. S. Schwartz, "Immunodeficiency and the Pathogenesis of Lymphoma and Leukemia," *Seminars in Hemotology* 15, no. 2 (1978): 117-138.
2. R. Hoover and J. F. Fraumeni, "Risk of Cancer in Renal Transplant Recipients," *Lancet* 2 (1973): 55-57.

Introduction

1. Lee Edson, "The Cancer Rip-Off," *Science Digest,* September 1974.
2. *Wall Street Journal,* October 24, 1978.
3. National Cancer Institute, *Cancer Prevention Research Summary-Viruses,* NIH Pub. No. 84-2612, February 1984, 1.
4. *Statistical Abstract of the United States,* U.S. Dept. of Commerce, Bureau of the Census, 1991.
5. *U.S. News & World Report,* August 20, 1984, 52.
6. *Consumer Digest,* January/February 1984.
7. John C. Bailar III, "Progress Against Cancer?," *New England Journal of Medicine* 314, no. 19 (May 8, 1986): 1226-32.
8. *New York Times,* November 27, 1984, C-1.
9. "The Cancer Watch," *U.S. News & World Report,* February 15, 1988, 12-13.
10. "The Cancer Sanction," *London Weekend Guardian,* September 29-30, 1990, 12.
11. American Cancer Society, *Cancer Facts and Figures—1990,* 3.
12. *New York Times.*
13. Ibid.
14. American Cancer Society, 8.
15. Ruth Rosenbaum, "Cancer, Inc.," *New Times,* November 25, 1977, 39.
16. U.S. General Accounting Office. "Cancer Patient Survival: What Progress Has Been Made?," Washington, D.C., March 1987.
17. Ralph W. Moss, *The Cancer Industry: Unraveling the Politics,* (New York: Paragon House, 1989), 22.
18. American Cancer Society, 3.
19. Ibid.
20. American Cancer Society, "Cancer Statistics—1990" in *Ca-A Cancer Journal for Clinicians* 40, no. 1 (January/February 1990): 9-10.

21. Ibid., p. 18.
22. American Cancer Society, *Cancer Facts and Figures*, p. 9.
23. Ibid, p. 14.
24. American Cancer Society, *Ca-A Cancer Journal for Clinicians* 41, no. 1 (January/February 1991): 36.
25. Ibid.
26. Bailar.
27. Ibid.
28. National Cancer Institute, p. 10.
29. *U.S. News & World Report.*
30. W. B. Cecil, *Textbook of Medicine*, (New York: Saunders Co., 1988), 1088.
31. Thomas Maugh and Jean L. Marx, *Seeds of Destruction: The Science Report on Cancer Research*, (New York: Plenum Publishing Corp., 1975).
32. R. Figlin, "Intracranial Recurrence of Carcinoma After Complete Surgical Resection of Non-Small Cell Lung Cancer," *NEJM* 318 (May 19, 1988): 1303.
33. P. Rubin, *Clinical Oncology for Medical Students. A Multidisciplinary Approach*, 6th ed. (New York and Rochester: ACS and the University of Rochester School of Medicine and Dentistry, 1983).
34. K. Shafer et. al., *Medical-Surgical Nursing*, (St. Louis: The C. V. Mosby Company, 1958), 597-98.
35. Hayes Martin, "The Case for Prophylactic Neck Dissection," *Ca-A Cancer Journal for Clinicians* 40, no. 4 (July/August 1990): 245-51.
36. Ibid.
37. W. Phipps et al., *Medical-Surgical Nursing*, (St. Louis: The C. V. Mosby Company, 1983), 1285.
38. Ibid., 1401
39. D. Lazovich et al., "Underutilization of Breast Conserving Surgery and Radiation Therapy Among Women with Stage I or II Breast Cancer," *Journal of the American Medical Association* 200 (December 25, 1991): 3433
40. Patricia Ganz, "Treatment Options for Breast Cancer Beyond Survival," *NEJM* 320, (April 23, 1992): 1147.
41. Lazovich.
42. W. Whitmore, "Management of Clinically Localized Cancer: An Unresolved Problem," *JAMA* 200 (May 20, 1993): 2070-72.
43. C. Fleming et al., "A Decision Analysis of Alternative Treatment Strategies for Clinically Localized Prostate Cancer," *JAMA* 200 (May 20, 1993): 2050-59.
44. R. Cittes, "Carcinoma of the Prostate," *NEJM* 324 (January 24, 1991): 230-3.
45. L. Grace et al, "An Assessment of Radical Prostatectomy: Time Trends, Geographic Variation and Outcomes," *JAMA* 200 (May 20, 1993): 2033-34.
46. J. Tobias, "Clinical Practice of Radiotherapy," *Lancet* 339 (January 18, 1992): 159.
47. Ibid.
48. Michael A. Weiner, *Maximum Immunity* (New York: Pocket Books, 1987), 183.
49. Woods, *Medical Surgical Nursing*, (Philadelphia: Lippincott, 1986), 236.
50. P. Woolf et al., "Hypothalmic-Pituitary Dysfunction After Radiation for Brain Tumors," *NEJM* 328 (January 14, 1993): 87.
51. S. Hancock et al., "Thyroid Diseases After Treatment of Hodgkin's Disease," *NEJM* 325 (August 29, 1991): 599.
52. A. Skolnick, "Primate Study Suggests Pentobarbital May Help Protect the Brain During Radiation Therapy," *JAMA* 264 (August 1, 1990): 557.

53. J. Neglia et al., "Second Neoplasms After Acute Lymphoblastic Leukemia in Childhood" *NEJM* 325 (November 7, 1991): 1330.
54. E. Row and M. Baruch, "Tumors of the Brain and Nervous System After Radiotherapy in Childhood," *NEJM* 319, no. 16 (October 20, 1988): 1038.
55. Ibid.
56. J. Boice et al., "Cancer in the Contralateral Breast After Radiotherapy for Breast Cancer," *NEJM* 326 (March 19, 1992): 781-85.
57. R. Curtis et al., "Risk of Leukemia After Chemotherapy and Radiation Treatment for Breast Cancer," *NEJM* 326 (June 25, 1992): 1745.
58. J. Cairns, "The Treatment of Diseases and the War Against Cancer," *Scientific American* Vol. 253 (November 1985) 51-9.
59. Ibid.
60. *Physicians' Desk Reference,* (New Jersey: Medical Economics Co., 1990), 1164.
61. *New York Times,* November 30, 1984, B-10.
62. *Physicians' Desk Reference,* 1166.
63. Ibid., 1163, col. 3 and 1790, col. 1.
64. Ibid., 572.
65. Ibid.
66. Moss, 87.
67. *Physicians' Desk Reference,* 1790.
68. Moss, 77.
69. *Physicians' Desk Reference,* 766.
70. Ibid.
71. Cecil, 1088.
72 *Physicians' Desk Reference,* 753.
73. Ibid., 755.
74. M. Mart et al., "Comparison of the 5-hydroxytryptamine 3 Antagonist Ondansetron with High Dose Metoclopramide in the Control of Cisplatin-induced Emesis," *NEJM* (March 22, 1990): 816.
75. Ibid.
76. *Is Cancer Curable?,* (California: Health Research Foundation, 1962), 65.
77. Hardin B. Jones, *"A Report on Cancer,"* presented to the American Cancer Society's 11th Annual Science Writers' Conference, New Orleans, Louisiana, March 7, 1969.
78. Ibid.
79. Ibid.
80. Ibid.
81. Moss, 33.
82. Ruth Rosenbaum, interview with Dr. E. Cuyler Hammond in *New Times,* 40.
83. *Lancet,* December 1975.
84. Cairns.

One: *Origins of the Alternative Therapy Movement*

1. J. W. Fell, *A Treatise on Cancer,* (London: John Churchill, 1975).
2. Maurice Natenberg, *The Cancer Blackout,* (Los Angeles: Cancer Control Society, 1974), 41.
3. W. B. Coley, *Archives of Surgery* 13, (December 1926): 780-836.
4. H. Nauts, "Bacterial Vaccine Therapy of Cancer," *Dev. Biol. Stan.* 38, (1977).
5. Natenberg, 78.

6. Natenberg, 80.
7. J. E. White, "Report on 100 Pathologically Proven Cases of Malignancy Treated by a Specific Antiserum," reprinted in *The Microbiology of Cancer*, (San Diego: The Livingston-Wheeler Medical Clinic, 1977), 297-303.
8. M. J. Scott, "Clinical Experiences with Carcinoma," *Irish Journal of Cancer* 3, no. 9 (1926): 1-6.
9. M. J. Scott, "The Parasitic Origin of Carcinoma," *Northwest Medicine* 24 (1925): 162-166.
10. T. J. Glover, Report on 200 Cases of Cancer Treated with Glover's Serum, *Philadelphia North American*, (June 9, 1924).
11. Ibid.
12. Ibid.
13. *New York Times*, June 10, 1924.
14. J. M. Wainwright, Corroboration of Cancer Remissions via Tissue Samples Received at the State Hospital for the Study of Malignant Diseases, Buffalo, New York, 1930.
15. E. L'Esperance, "Studies in Hodgkin's Disease." *Annals of Surgery* 93, (1931): 162-168.
16. G. Mazet, "Etude bactériologique sur la maladie d'Hodgkin," *Montpellier Médicine*, (Juillet/Aout 1941).
17. Mori Nello, "Virus filtrabili e cancro secondo la mia ipotesi della loro nature micetica," *Progresso Medico* 6 (1950): 3-31.
18. Francisco Duran Reynals, "Neoplastic Infections and Cancer," *American Journal of Medicine* 3, no. 4 (1950): 440-511.
19. V. Wuerthele-Caspe and Roy Allen, "Microorganisms Associated with Neoplasms," *New York Microscopical Society Bulletin* 2 (1948): 2-31.
20. White.
21. Arie Audier, *Die Medizinische* 40 (1959): 1860-64.
22. Judith Glassman, *The Cancer Survivors*, (New York: Dial Press, 1983), 218.
23. American Cancer Society, *Dubious Cancer Treatment*, (1991), 47.
24. Robert Houston, *Repression and Reform in the Evaluation of Alternative Cancer Therapies*, (Washington, D.C.: Project Cure, 1989), 7.
25. Ed Griffin, *World Without Cancer*, (California: American Media, 1977) 23.
26. Ibid.

Two: *Gerson's Diet Therapy*

1. F. Sauerbach, *Das War Mein Leiben*, (Kindler und Schiermeyer Verlag: Bad Woerischoffen, 1951), 363-71.
2. American Cancer Society, *The Gerson Method of Treatment of Cancer*, (August 1972).
3. F. Sauerbach and M. Gerson, "Ueber Versuche, schwere Formen der Tuberkulose diatetische Behandlugen zu beeinflussen," *Muench. Medizinische Wochenschrift* 2, no. 1 (1926).
4. E. Urbach and E. B. Le Winn, *Skin Diseases, Nutrition and Metabolism* (New York: Grune and Stratton, 1946), 4, 65-67, 530-37. (Presents an overview of Gerson's clinical TB trials.)
5. Max Gerson, *Muench, Medizinische Wochenschrift* 23 (1930).
6. Max Gerson, *A Cancer Therapy* (California: Gerson Institute, 1986), 31-32.

7. F. R. White, *Journal of the National Cancer Institute* 5 (1944): 43.
8. H. P. Rush et al., *Cancer Research Journal* 5, (1945): 431.
9. C. D. Larsen and W. E. Heston, *Journal of the National Cancer Institute* 6, (1945) 31.
10. A Tannenbaum, *American Journal of Cancer* 38 (1940): 335.
11. Ibid.
12. Otto Warburg, *The Prime Cause and Prevention of Cancer* (Würzburg, Germany: Konrad Triltsch, 1969). (Contains an overview of Warburg's research and the scientific reference of his published articles.)
13. Ibid.
14. Gerson, *A Cancer Therapy*, 89-91, 163-65.
15. Ibid., 63-64.
16. Ibid., 196, 211.
17. Ibid., 407.
18. Ibid., 191.
19. P. Lechner and I. Kroenberger, "Experiences with the Use of Dietary Therapy in Surgical Oncology," *Tropical Nutritional Medicine* 2, band 15 (April 1990).
20. Testimony given before a Subcommittee of the United States Senate, 79th Congress, 2nd session, on Bill S.1875, July 1-3, 1946.
21. Ibid.
22. Ibid.
23. John Gunther Sr., *Death Be Not Proud,* (New York: Doubleday, 1949).
24. Ibid.
25. Ibid.
26. *Physicians' Desk Reference,* (New Jersey: Medical Economics, 1990) 1216, col. 2.
27. Ibid.
28. Testimony given before a Subcommittee of the United States Senate, 79th Congress, 2nd session, on Bill S.1875, July 1-3, 1946.
29. Ibid.
30. Ibid.
31. Ibid.
32. Ibid.
33. Ibid.
34. Ibid.
35. Ibid.
36. Ibid.
37. Gunther.
38. Stephen P. Strickland, "Integration of Medical Research and Health Politics," *Science* (September 17, 1971).
39. "Gerson's Cancer Treatment" (editorial), *JAMA* 132 (1946): 645-46.
40. National Cancer Institute: Statement on Gerson Therapy, May 11, 1988.
41. Letter to the ACS from General Counsel, New York County Medical Society, March 27, 1989.
42. Gerson, *A Cancer Therapy,* 251-389.
43. Ibid.
44. *Ca-A Cancer Journal for Clinicians* 40, no. 4 (July/August 1990): 255.
45. Ibid.
46. Ibid., 256.
47. Ibid., 253.

48. Ibid., 255.
49. A. Reed, N. Jame, and K. Sikora. *Lancet* 336, no. 8716 (September 15, 1990): 677-78.
50. J. Lowell, "The Gerson Clinic," *Nutritional Forum* 3 (1989): 9-12.
51. Ibid.
52. Lancet.
53. Ibid.
54. P. Lechner and I. Kroenberger, "Experiences with the Use of Dietary Therapy in Surgical Oncology," *Tropical Nutritional Medicine* 2, band 15 (April 1990).
55. Ibid.
56. Ibid.
57. Saul Green, "A Critique of the Rationale for Cancer Treatment with Coffee Enemas and Diet," *JAMA* 268, no. 22 (December 9, 1992): 3224-27.

Three: *The Livingston Therapy*

1. Kenneth C. Forror, Personal communication, The Livingston Foundation Medical Center, San Diego, May 1992.
2. Virginia Livingston, Curriculum Vitae, The Livingston Foundation Medical Center.
3. Ibid.
4. American Cancer Society. Statement on Virginia Livingston, June 7, 1989.
5. V. Livingston, E. Jackson, and W. L. Smith, "Some Aspects of the Microbiology of Cancer," *Journal of the American Medical Women's Association* 10, no. 8 (August 1955): 261-266.
6. V. Livingston, "Cultural Properties and Pathogenicity of Certain Microorganisms Obtained from Various Proliferative and Neoplastic Diseases," *American Journal of the Medical Sciences* 220 (December 1950): 638-648.
7. V. Livingston, et al., "Microbiology of Cancer, Neoplastic Infection of Men and Animals," Atti Del VI Congresso Internazionale Di Microbiologica, Roma, Vol. 6, Sez XVII (September 1953) 3-9.
8. V. Livingston and E. Jackson, "A Specified Type of Organism Cultivated from Malignancy: Bacteriology and Proposed Classification," *Annals of the New York Academy of Sciences* 174, art. 2 (October 1970): 636-54.
9. Edmond G. Addeo, *The Conquest of Cancer,* (New York: Franklin Watts, 1984): 69-70.
10. Ibid.
11. Ibid., 97.
12. W. M. Crofton, *The Cure of Acute and Chronic Infections by Active Immunization,* (London: John Bale Medical Publishers Ltd., 1939).
13. Addeo, 97.
14. Ibid., 47.
15. Ibid.
16. V. Livingston and E. A. Jackson. An Experimental Biologic Approach to the Treatment of Neoplastic Diseases," *Journal of the American Medical Women's Association* 20, no. 5 (May 1965): 449-52.
17. E. Jackson, "Ultraviolet Spectrogramic Microscope Studies of Rous Sarcoma Virus Cultured in Cell-free Medium," *Annals of the New York Academy of Sciences* 174, Art. 2 (October 30, 1970): 765-81.

18. "Nutrition, the Changing Scene," *Lancet* (April 16, 1983) from W. Bollag, *Vitamin A and Retionoids: From Nutrition to Pharmacotherapy in Dermatology and Oncology.*

19. I. C. Diller, et al., "Tumor Incidence in ICR/Albino Male Mice Injected with Organisms Cultured from Malignant Mouse Tissues," *Growth* 38 (1974): 507-17.

20. F. B. Seibert et al., "Decrease in Spontaneous Tumors by Vaccinating C3H Mice with an Homologous Bacterial Vaccine," IRCS International Communications System, March 1973.

21. American Cancer Society, *Statement on Virginia Livingston,* November 1972.

22. Ibid.

23. V. Djurovic and G. Decroix, "Five Years of Active Nonspecific Immunotherapy With a Transformed Mycobacterium in Surgically-Treated Primary Lung Cancers. One to Three Years of Post-Operative Follow-Up, *Société Français de Radiologie Medicale* 59, no. 11 (1978): 651-54.

24. Addeo, 18.

25. National Cancer Institute, *Cancer Prevention Research Summary-Viruses,* NIH Pub. No. 84-2612 (February 1984): 1.

26. Personal correspondence, National Cancer Institute, Bethesda, Maryland, June 22, 1987.

27. M. F. Barile et al., "Isolation of Mycoplasma from Leukemic Bone Marrow and Blood by Direct Culture," *Journal of the National Cancer Institute* 36 (1966): 161.

28. Joseph Tully, "Mycoplasma in Leukemic and Nonleukemic Mice," *Annals of the New York Academy of Sciences,* (July 28, 1967): 345-52.

29. William Murphy et al., "Isolation of Mycoplasma from Leukemic and Nonleukemic Patients," *JNCI* 45, no. 2 (August 1970).

30. Alva H. Johnson, Professor of Microbiology, University of Eastern Virginia Medical School, personal communication, May 22, 1992.

31. American Cancer Society, *Cancer Journal for Clinicians* 40, no. 2 (March/April 1990).

32. Johnson.

33. V. Livingston, "Some Cultural, Immunological, and Biochemical Properties of Progenitor Cryptocides," *Transactions of the New York Academy of Sciences* 36, series II, no. 6 (June 1974): 569-82.

34. *Merck Manual,* 15th Edition, (New Jersey: Merck & Co., Inc., 1987) 1685, 1744-45.

35. E. R. Pinckney, *The Patient's Guide to Medical Tests,* (New York: Facts on File, 1986) 268.

36. H. Cohen and A. Strammp, "Bacterial Synthesis of Substance Similar to HCG," *Proceedings of the Society for Experimental Biology and Medicine* 152, no. 3 (July 1976).

37. H. F. Acevedo et al., "HCG in Cancer Cells I. Identification in *in vitro* and *in vivo* Ca-Cell Systems," in H. E. Neiburgs, ed. *Detection and Prevention of Cancer* part 2, vol. 1 (New York: Marcel Dekker, Inc., 1976) 957-63.

38. L. McManus et al., "Human Chorionic Gonadotropin in Human Neoplastic Cells," *Cancer Research* 36 (1976): 3476.

39. W. D. Van Beek, L. A. Smets, and P. Emmelot, "Changed Surface Glycoprotein as a Marker of Malignancy in Human Leukemic Cells," *Nature* 253 (1975): 457-60.

194 *Notes*

40. A. Whyte and Y. W. Loke, "Increased Sialylation of Surface Glycopeptides of Human Trophoblast Compared with Fetal Cells from the Same Conceptus," *Journal of Experimental Medicine* 148 (1978) 1087-92.
41. "The Quest for a Cancer Vaccine," *Newsweek,* October 19, 1992.
42. Barrie R. Cassileth et al., "Survival and Quality of Life Among Patients Receiving Unproven as Compared with Conventional Cancer Therapy," *New England Journal of Medicine* 324 (April 25, 1991): 1180.
43. Personal communication, The Livingston Foundation Medical Center, May 1, 1992.
44. *NEJM,* 1180.
45. "New Drug from an Old Preparation Offers Hope Against Bladder Cancer," *New York Times,* August 9, 1990, B-10.
46. Ibid.
47. Ibid.
48. Johnson.

Four: *Hydrazine Sulfate*

1. Joseph Gold, "Use of Hydrazine Sulfate in Terminal or Preterminal Cancer Patients: Results of IND Study in 84 Evaluable Patients," *Oncology* 32 (1975): 1-10.
2. Ralph Moss, *The Cancer Industry,* (New York: Paragon House, 1989), 196.
3. Jeff Kamen, "Hope, Heartbreak and Horror," *OMNI,* (September 1993).
4. Joseph Gold, "Hydrazine Sulfate: A Current Perspective," *Nutrition and Cancer* 9, nos. 2, 3 (1987).
5. S. Robins, *Textbook of Pathology,* (Philadelphia: Saunders, 1957).
6. G. Costa et al., "Weight Loss and Cachexia in Lung Cancer," *Nutrition and Cancer* 2 (1980): 98-103.
7. O. Warburg, *The Prime Cause and Prevention of Cancer,* (Würzburg, German: Konrad Triltsch, 1969).
8. P. D. Ray, "Inhibition of Gluconeogenesis by Hydrazine," *Fed Proc* 28 (1969): 411.
9. Gold.
10. Ibid.
11. M. Ochoa et al., "Trial of Hydrazine Sulfate in Patients with Cancer," *Cancer Chemotherapy Report* 58 (1975): 1151-54.
12. Moss, 193.
13. J. F. Seits et al., "Experimental and Clinical Data of Antitumor Action of Hydrazine Sulfate," *Problems of Oncology,* 21 (1975).
14. Ibid.
15. V. A. Filov et al., "Results of Clinical Evaluation of Hydrazine Sulfate," *Vopr Onkol* 36, no. 6 (1990): 721-26.
16. American Cancer Society, *Facts and Figures,* 1990.
17. Filov.
18. Ibid.
19. Ibid.
20. Ibid.
21. M. Gersanovich, "Hydrazine Sulfate in Late Stage Cancer: Completion of Initial Clinical Trials in 225 Evaluable Patients," *Proceedings of the American Association for Cancer Research,* (Baltimore: Cancer Research Inc., 1979).

22. R. Chlebowski et al., "Influence of Hydrazine Sulfate on Abnormal Carbohydrate Metabolism in Cancer Patients with Weight Loss," *Cancer Research* 44 (1984) 857-61.
23. Ibid.
24. R. Chlebowski et al., "Influence of Hydrazine Sulfate on Food Intake and Weight Maintenance in Patients with Cancer," *Proc Am Soc Clin Oncol* 4, (1985): 265.
25. R. Chlebowski et al., "Hydrazine Sulfate in Cancer Patients with Weight Loss," *Cancer* 59 (1987) 406-410.
26. J. L. Mulshine et al. "Treatment of Non-Small Cell Lung Cancer," *Journal of Clinical Oncology* 4 (1968): 1704-15.
27. R. Chlebowski et al., "Hydrazine Sulfate Influence on Nutritional Status and Survival in NSCLC," *J. Clin Oncol.* 8, no. 1, (January 1990): 9-15.
28. Ibid.
29. D. M. Finkelstein et al., "Long-Term Survivors in Metastatic NSCLC: An Eastern Cooperative Oncology Group Study," *J Clin Oncol* 4 (1986): 702-9.
30. Chlebowski.
31. J. Tayek et al., "Effect of Hydrazine Sulfate on Whole-Body Protein Breakdown Measured by C-Lysine Metabolism in Lung Cancer Patients," *Lancet* (August 1, 1987).
32. Kamen.
33. Ibid.
34. Ibid.
35. Ibid.
36. Chlebowski.
37. Ibid.

Five: *Immuno-Augmentative Therapy*

1. *Immuno-Augmentative Therapy*, Freeport, Bahamas, 29.
2. Curriculum Vitae, *Immuno-Augmentative Therapy*.
3. Ibid.
4. Ibid., 22.
5. Ralph Moss, *The Cancer Industry*, (New York: Paragon House, 1989), 243.
6. IAT Center, (1985).
7. E. Creagan et al., "Failure of High-Dose Vitamin C Therapy to Benefit Patients with Advanced Cancer," *New England Journal of Medicine* 301 (September 27, 1979), 687-90.
8. R. G. Houston, *Repression and Reform in the Evaluation of Alternative Cancer Therapies*, (Washington, D.C.: Project Cure, Inc., 1989), 27.
9. Ibid.
10. Ibid.
11. Congressional Public Hearing before Congressman Guy V. Molinari, "A Hearing on the Immuno-Augmentative Therapy of Dr. Lawrence Burton," New York: Chesapeake Reporting Service, January 15, 1986, 168.
12. Ibid., 169.
13. Ibid., 171.
14. Ibid., 172.
15. Ibid., 97.
16. American Cancer Society, *Dubious Cancer Treatment*, 1991, 65.
17. Ibid., 66.

18. Ibid.
19. Ibid.
20. B. Stone, FDA Issues Alert Against Dangerous Cancer Remedy, FDA Talk Paper T86-60. Rockville, Maryland, August 1986.
21. Congressional Hearing, 38-39.
22. Alan Anderson, "The Politics of Cancer: How Do You Get the Medical Establishment to Listen?," *New York,* July 29, 1974, 45.
23. Ibid.
24. Ibid., 46.
25. Ibid.
26. *60 Minutes*, CBS Television Network 12, no. 36, May 18, 1980.
27. Moss, 249.
28. S. Insalaco et al., "Isolation of HTLV-III from Samples of Serum Proteins Given to Cancer Patients," *Morbidity, Mortality Weekly Report* 34, (1985): 489-91.
29. Ibid.
30. Ibid.
31. Virginia H. Knauer, Special Adviser to President Reagan for Consumer Affairs; Speech delivered at the National Press Club to the National Health Fraud Conference, Washington, D.C., September 11, 1985.
32. Guy Molinari, Congressional Hearing.
33. IAT Sera Screening report, Pierce County Blood Bank, Tacoma, Washington, in *Health Consciousness* 7, no. 4 (August 1986).
34. "A Consumer Guide to Testing," *U.S. News & World Report,* April 20, 1987, 61.
35. Gary Null, "The Vendetta Against Dr. Burton," *Penthouse,* March 1986.
36. *Health Consciousness,* 7.
37. Null.
38. *The Birmingham News,* November 7, 1985.
39. *Health Consciousness,* 7.
40. Houston, 24.
41. Donald R. Steele, "HTLV-III Antibodies in Human Immune y-Globulin," Letter to the Editor, *Journal of the American Medical Association* 255, no. 5 (February 7, 1986).
42. Ibid.
43. *Health Consciousness,* 7.
44. G. A. Curt, "Warning on Immunoaugmentative Therapy," *NEJM* 311, (1984): 859.
45. *Health Consciousness,* 7.
46. M. Goldsmith, "Blood Bank Officials Hope Donor Altruism Will Pass New [Anti-HCV] Test," *JAMA* 263 (April 4, 1990) 1749.
47. J. M. Starkey et al., "Markers for Transfusion-Transmitted Disease in Different Groups of Blood Donors," *JAMA* 262 (December 22, 1989): 3452.
48. M. Goldsmith.
49. H. Alter et al., "Detection of Antibody to Hepatitis C Virus in Prospectively Followed Transfusion Recipients with Acute Chronic Non-A, Non-B Hepatitis," *NEJM* 321 (November 30, 1989): 1494.
50. Congressional Hearing, 53-54.
51. Ibid.
52. "Diagnostic and Therapeutic Technology Assessment," *JAMA* 259, no. 23 (June 17, 1988): 3478.
53. G. Young, "Disputed Bahamas Cancer Clinic Reopens," *Newsday,* March 11, 1986.

54. B. R. Cassileth et al., Report on a Survey of Patients Receiving Immuno-Augmentative Therapy," Philadelphia: University of Pennsylvania Cancer Center, 1987.
55. Ibid.
56. Ibid.
57. Robert Houston, "Analysis of a Survey of Patients on Immuno-Augmentative Therapy," Iowa: People Against Cancer, 5-6.
58. Ibid., 3-6.
59. Ibid.
60. L. Burton, "Peritoneal Mesothelioma," *Quantum Medicine* 1, no. 1, 2 (January-April 1988).
61. Ibid.
62. Ibid.

Six: *Vitamin C Therapy*

1. L. Pauling and E. Cameron, *Cancer and Vitamin C*, (New York: W. W. Norton, 1979).
2. Ibid.
3. J. Paradowski, Biographical note in Linus Pauling, *How to Live Longer and Feel Better*, (New York: Avon Books, 1986.)
4. John Horgan, "Profile: Linus C. Pauling Stubbornly Ahead of His Time." *Scientific American*, March 1993, 36-40.
5. Ibid.
6. J. A. Lind, *A Treatise of Scurvy*, (Edinburgh: Sands, Murray and Cochrane, Edinburgh University Press, 1953).
7. H. Appelbaum, "Vitamin C and Cancer," Dissertation for M.D. degree, University of Zurich, 1937.
8. Pauling, *Cancer and Vitamin C*, 124.
9. Ibid.
10. Ibid.
11. Ibid.
12. Ibid.
13. E. Cameron and L. Pauling, "Supplemental Ascorbate in the Supportive Treatment of Cancer: Prolongation of Survival Times in Terminal Human Cancer." *Proceedings of the National Academy of Sciences* 73 (1976) 3685-89.
14. Ibid.
15. F. Morishige and A. Murata, "Prolongation of Survival Times in Terminal Human Cancer by Administration of Supplemental Ascorbate," *Journal of the International Academy of Preventive Medicine* 5 (1978): 47-52.
16. S. Bram, "Vitamin C Preferential Toxicity for Malignant Melanoma Cells," *Nature* (1980): 284.
17. E. Creagan and C. Moertel, "Failure of High-Dose Vitamin C Therapy to Benefit Patients with Advanced Cancer," *New England Journal of Medicine* 301 (September 27, 1979): 687-90.
18. Ibid.
19. Ibid.
20. Ibid.
21. Pauling, *How to Live Longer and Feel Better*, 233.
22. Cancer Research 35 (1975): 3075-83.
23. American Cancer Society, *Dubious Cancer Treatment*, 1991, 81.

cat

24. Pauling, *Cancer and Vitamin C*, 142
25. American Cancer Society, Statement on Vitamin C, 1981.
26. Ibid.
27. C. G. Moertel et al., "High-Dose Vitamin C versus Placebo in the Treatment of Patients with Advanced Cancer Who Have Had No Prior Chemotherapy," *NEJM* 312 (1985): 137-41.
28. Ibid.
29. M. A. Weiner, *Maximum Immunity*, (New York: Simon & Schuster, 1987), 192.
30. Pauling, *How to Live Longer and Feel Better*, 313.
31. Ibid., 234.
32. Ullica Segerstrale, "Beleaguering the Cancer Establishment," *Science* 255 (January 31, 1992): 614.
33. Ibid.
34. L. Pauling and Z. Herman, "Criteria for the Validity of Clinical Trials of Treatments of Cohorts of Cancer Patients based on the Hardin Jones Principle," *Proceedings of the National Academy of Sciences* 86 (1989): 6835-37.
35. Segerstrale, 615.
36. M. Barinaga, "Vitamin C Gets a Little Respect," *Science* 254 (October 18, 1991): 374.
37. Ibid., 375.
38. M. E. Poydock, "Inhibiting Effect of Dehydroascorbic Acid on Cell Division in Ascites Tumors in Mice," *Exp. Cell Biol.* 50 (1982): 34-38.
39. H. Riordan, "High Dose Vitamin C in the Treatment of a Patient with Adenocarcinoma of the Kidney," *Journal of Orthomolecular Medicine* 5 (1990): 5-7.
40. Barinaga, 375.
41. *Physicians' Desk Reference*, 44th edition, (New Jersey: Medical Economics, 1990) 573-574.
42. S. Marcus, "Severe Hypovitaminosis C Occurring as the Result of Adoptive Immunotherapy with High Dose Interleukin 2 and Lymphokine-activated Killer Cells," *Cancer Research* 47 (1987).
43. Barinaga, 374.
44. Ibid.
45. B. Frei, "Ascorbate: the Most Effective Antioxidant in Human Blood Plasma," *Adv. Exp. Med. Biol.* 264 (1990): 155-63.
46. Barinaga, 375.
47. R. F. Cathcart, "Vitamin C Treatment Protocol for AIDS," in Weiner, 335.
48. S. Fukushima, "Promoting Effects of Sodium L-Ascorbate on Two-stage Urinary Bladder Carcinogenesis in Rats," *Cancer Research* 43 (1983): 4454-57.
49. *Physicians' Desk Reference*, 915.

Seven: *Laetrile*

1. *Gazette Medicale de Paris* 37 (1845): 577-82.
2. American Cancer Society, Statement on Laetrile, July 1990.
3. Ibid.
4. Ralph Moss, *The Cancer Industry*, (New York: Paragon House 1989), 140.
5. Mark McCarty, "Burying Caesar: An Analysis of the Laetrile Problem," *Triton Times*, University of California, San Diego, Nov. 24-26, 1975.

6. L. W. Wattenburg, "Inhibition of Carcinogenic Effects of Polycyclic Hydrocarbons by Benzyl Isothiocyanate and related Compounds," *Journal of the National Cancer Institute* 58 (1977): 395-98.

7. R. E. Heikkila and F. S. Cabbat, "The Prevention of Alloxan-induced Diabetes by Amygdalin," *Life Sciences* 27 (1980): 659-62.

8. Arthur T. Harris, "Possible Palliative Value of Laetrile in Human Cancer. A Preliminary Report (1953)," in Kittler, *Laetrile: Nutritional Control for Cancer,* (Denver: Royal Publications, 1978).

9. H. H. Beard, *A New Approach to the Conquest of Cancer and Heart Diseases,* (Los Angeles: Cancer Book House, 1962).

10. Ettore Guidetti, "Preliminary Observations on Cancer Cases Treated With A Cyanogenetic Glycuronoside," *Acta Unio Internationalis Contra Cancrum,* 11, no. 2 (1955) 156-59.

11. Ibid.

12. Cancer Commission of the California Medical Association. Report on Laetrile in *California Medicine,* (April 1953).

13. John W. Budd, Report on Laetrile, California Advisory Council, Department of Public Health, 1963, App. 4, 1-2.

14. Ed Griffin, *World Without Cancer,* (California: American Media, 1974), 32-33.

15. Griffin, 27.

16. K. N. Shafer et al., *Medical Surgical Nursing,* (St. Louis: C. V. Mosby Co. 1958) 217.

17. Griffin, 28.

18. Griffin, 31.

19. Manuel Navarro, "The Mechanism of Action and Therapeutics of Laetrile in Cancer," *Journal of Philippine Medicine* 33 (1957) 620-27.

20. Manuel Navarro et al., "Five Years Experience with Laetrile Therapy in Advanced Cancer," *Acta Unio Internationalis Contra Cancrum* 15 (1959), 209-21.

21. N. Tasca, "Clinical Observations on the Therapeutic Effects of a Cyanogenetic Glucoronoside in Cases of Human Malignant Neoplasms," *Gazetta Medica Italiana* 118 (April 1959) 153-59.

22. John Morrone, M.D., "Chemotherapy of Inoperable Cancer. Preliminary Report of 10 Cases Treated with Laetrile," *Experimental Medicine and Surgery* no. 4, (1962).

23. Ibid.

24. Ibid.

25. Ralph Moss, *The Cancer Industry* (New York: Paragon House, 1989) 158-59.

26. Kanematsu Sugiura, "A Summary of the Effect of Amygdalin Upon Spontaneous Mammary Tumors in Mice," Sloan-Kettering Institute report, June 13, 1973.

27. Glenn D. Kittler, *Laetrile: Nutritional Control for Cancer,* (Denver: Royal Publications, 1978), 109.

28. Moss, 175.

29. American Cancer Society, Statement on Laetrile, December 18, 1992.

30. Moss, 176-77.

31. Southern Research Institute, Birmingham, Alabama, for the National Cancer Institute, December 3, 1973.

32. Carl Baker, Director NCI, Letter to Congressman Edwin W. Edwards, January 26, 1971, referring to Studies Conducted by the Scind Laboratories, University of San Francisco, October 10, 1968.
33. P. G. Reitnauer, "Prolongation of Life in Tumor-Bearing Mice by Bitter Almonds," *Arch. Geschwulstforsch* 42, no. 4 (1974): 135-37.
34. J. E. Craige, "Of Canine Cancer and Vitamin B-17: Veterinarian Takes a Look at Laetrile," *The Choice* 2, no. 5 (June 1976).
35. "NCI Finds Laetrile Ineffective," *Science News* 119 (May 9, 1981) 293.
36. American Cancer Society.
37. Ibid.
38. Ibid.
39. Ibid.
40. "Laetrile Study," *Star Ledger,* Newark, New Jersey, June 7, 1981.
41. Michael Culbert, "Rebuttal to ACS Laetrile Denunciation," *Townsend Letter for Doctors,* (June 1992): 488-92.
42. Ibid.

Eight: *Burzynski's Antineoplastons*

1. Saul Green, Ph. D. "'Antineoplastons' An Unproved Cancer Therapy," *Journal of the American Medical Association* 267, no. 21 (June 3, 1992): 2924.
2. American Cancer Society Response System: Antineoplastons, no. 8016, July 2, 1991.
3. G. Ungar and S. R. Burzynski, "Detection of a Behavior Inducing Peptide from Brains of Trained Rats," *Fed. Proc.* 31 (1972): 398.
4. G. Ungar and S. R. Burzynski, "Isolation and Purification of Habituation Inducing Peptides from Brains of Trained Rats," *Fed. Proc.* 32 (1973): 367.
5. Green.
6. "Antineoplastons: An Investigational Cancer Therapy," *Townsend Letter for Doctors,* (February/March 1993).
7. Burzynski Research Institute brochure.
8. Ibid.
9. Ibid.
10. S. R. Burzynski et al., "Antineoplaston A in Cancer Therapy," *Physiology, Chemistry and Physics* 9 (1977): 485.
11. Ibid.
12. *Ca-A Cancer Journal for Clinicians* 36, no. 6 (1986).
13. "Articles and Monographs" of Stanislaw R. Burzynski M.D. in Burzynski Clinic, Houston, Texas.
14. S. R. Burzynski, "Antineoplastons: History of the Research," *Drugs Under Experimental and Clinical Research* Suppl. 1. (1986): 1-9.
15. S. R. Burzynski, *Drugs of the Future* 11 (1986): 679-88.
16. S. R. Burzynski, Speech to the 14th International Cancer Congress, Budapest, Hungary, 1986.
17. S. R. Burzynski and E. Kubove, *Drugs Under Experimental and Clinical Research* Suppl. 1, 13 (1987): 1-43.
18. Ibid.
19. S. R. Burzynski, E. Kubove and B. Burzinski, "Phase II Clinical Trials of Antineoplaston 10 and AS2-1 Infusions in Astrocytoma," 17th International Congress of Chemotherapy, Berlin, Germany, 1991.

20. Ibid.
21. Green, 2926.
22. D. Samid et al., "Phenylacetate: a Novel Nontoxic Inducer of Tumor Cell Differentiation," *Cancer Research* 52 (1992): 1988-92.
23. A. F. Lehner, S. R. Burzynski and L. B. Hendry, "3 Phenylacetylamino 2, 6-piperidinedione, a Naturally Occurring Peptide Analog with Apparent Antineoplastic Activity May Bind to DNA," *Drugs Under Experimental and Clinical Research,* Suppl. 1, 12 (1986): 57.
24. L. B. Hendry, T. G. Muldoon et al., "Stereochemical Modeling Studies of the Interaction of A-10 with DNA," *Drugs Under Experimental and Clinical Research,* Suppl. 1, 12 (1986).
25. "Antineoplastons: New Antitumor Agents Stir High Expectations," *Oncology News* 16, no. 4 (July/August 1990): 1.
26. Ibid.
27. Ibid.
28. Green.
29. Saul Green, Letter in *Journal of the American Medical Association* 269, no. 4 (January 27, 1993): 476.
30. "Antineoplastons: An Investigational Cancer Therapy," *Townsend Letter for Doctors* (February/March 1993): 150.
31. H. Tsuda and H. Hara, "The Anticancer Effect of Antineoplaston A-10 on Human Breast Cancer Serially Transplanted to Athymic Mice," *The Journal of Japan Society for Cancer Therapy* 25, no. 1 (January 20, 1990): 4.
32. *JAMA* 267, no. 21 (June 3, 1992): 2926-27.
33. Ibid.
34. Ibid.
35. Ibid.
36. H. Tsuda, written communication to Dr. S. R. Burzynski, June 1992 in *Townsend Letter for Doctors,* 152.
37. H. Tsuda, and H. Hara, *The Journal of Japan Society for Cancer Therapy* 25.
38. H. Tsuda et al., "The Inhibitory Effect of Combination Use of Antineoplaston-10 Injection with Small Dose CDDP on Cell and Tumor Growth of Human Hepatocellular Carcinoma," presented at the 17th International Congress of Chemotherapy, Berlin, Germany, 1991.
39. H. Tsuda, and H. Hara, *The Journal of Japan Society for Cancer Therapy* 25.
40. Ibid.
41. S. R. Burzynski, written communication to V. L. Narayanan, Ph. D., NCI, June 1984.
42. *Townsend Letter for Doctors,* 152.
43. W. Xu et al., "The Preliminary Antitumor Assay of Antineoplaston A-10 Against S-180 and the Effects on cAMP Levels in Tumor and Liver Tissues of Mice," *Department of Pharmacy Bulletin,* Jinan, People's Republic of China: Shandong Medical University, (1988).
44. T. G. Muldoon et al., "Inhibition of Spontaneous Mouse Mammary Tumor Development by Antineoplaston-10," *Drugs Under Experimental and Clinical Research* Suppl. 1, 13 (1987): 83-88.
45. American Cancer Society.
46. Ibid.
47. S. A. Shepartz, Ph. D., written communication to National Cancer Institute, July 9, 1992.

48. American Cancer Society.
49. *Discoveries in Medicine,* Mutual Benefit Life, Winter, 1991, 5.
50. Director of Antineoplaston Study Group at the Kurume Medical School, Letter in *Townsend Letter for Doctors,* 152.
51. S. R. Burzynski et al., "Phase II Clinical Trial of Antineoplastons A-10 and AS2-1 Infusions in Astrocytoma," *Recent Advances in Chemotherapy,* (Munich, Germany: Futuramed Publishers, 1992).
52. S. R. Burzynski et al., "Treatment of Hormonally Refractory Cancer of the Prostate with Antineoplaston AS2-1," *Drugs Under Experimental and Clinical Research* 16 (1990): 361.
53. M. R. Grever, M.D., Director of Developmental Therapeutics, written communication, National Cancer Institute, 1992.
54. M. J. Hawkings, M.D., Chief, Investigational Drug Branch, Cancer Therapy Evaluation Program, Division of Cancer Treatment, NCI, written communication, February 1992 in *JAMA* (June 3, 1992): 2927.
55. Lee Trombetta, personal communication, Burzynski Research Institute, July 29, 1993.
56. *Health Facts,* (March 1992).
57. Robert Houston, *Repression and Reform in the Evaluation of Alternative Cancer Therapies,* (Washington: Project Cure, 1989): 17-18.
58. Interview with Ralph Moss in *Health Facts,* 2-3.
59. Ibid.
60. *Houston Chronicle,* October 4, 1985.

Nine: *Hyperthermia*

1. R. Cavaliere et al., "Selective Heat Sensitivity of Cancer Cells," *Cancer* no. 20 (September 1967): 1351-81.
2. Y. Kida et al. "Hyperthermia of Metastatic Brain Tumor with Implant Heating System: Preliminary Clinical Results," *No Shinkei Geka* 6 (June 1990): 521-26.
3. J. Hahl et al., Laser Induced Hyperthermia in the Treatment of Liver Tumors," *Lasers Surg Med* 10, no. 4 (1990): 319-21.
4. T. Satou, "Warm Drug Solution Injected into Tumor Vessel May Enhance Antitumor Effect," *Gan To Kagaku Ryoho,* 178, pt. 2 (August 1990): 1763-77.
5. K. Kobayashi et al., "Clinical Effect of Intraperitoneal Hyperthermochemotherapy on the Survival Rate for Advanced Gastric Cancer Patients," *Gan To Kagaku Ryoho,* 178, pt. 2 (August 1990): 1617-21.
6. R. Lewis, "Cancer Treatments Go Hot and Cold," *Health,* (February 1988), 88.
7. Ibid.
8. H. Bicher et al., "Clinical Use of Regional Hyperthermia," in *Consensus on Hyperthermia for the 1990s,* (New York: Plenum Press, 1990).
9. J. B. Dubois, "Superficial Microwave-Induced Hyperthermia in the Treatment of Chest Wall Recurrences in Breast Cancer," *Cancer* 66, no. 5 (September 1, 1990): 848-52.
10. A. S. Mavrichev, "Whole-Body Artificial Controlled Hyperthermia and Hyperglycemia in the Combined Treatment of Metastatic Kidney Cancer," *Urol Nefrol* 3 (May/June 1990): 48-52.
11. A. Hayashi, "Honing in on Cancer Cells," *Technology Review* 96 (January 1993): 12.

Ten: *Hoxsey Method*

1. American Cancer Society Cancer Response System: Hoxsey Method Biomedical Center, July 15, 1991.
2. Ibid.
3. Ibid.
4. Ibid.
5. Ibid.
6. Ibid.
7. Morita Kazuyoshi et al., "A Desmutagenic Factor Isolated from Burdock," *Mutation Research* 129, (1984): 25-31.
8. A. Hoshi et al., "Antitumor Activity of Berberine Derivatives," *Japanese Journal of Cancer Research,* no. 67 (1976).
9. ACS.
10. T. Aoki et al., "Human Colorectal Carcinoma-Specific Glycoconjugates Detected by Pokeweed Mitogen Lectin," J *Histochem Cytochem* 41, no. 9 (September 1993): 1321-30.
11. K. Morikawa et al., "Recombinant Human IL-5 Augments Immunoglobulin Generation by Human B Lymphocytes in the Presence of IL-2," *Cell Immunology* 149, no. 2 (July 1993): 390-401.
12. D. Chauhan et al., "Regulation of c-jun Gene Expression in Human T Lymphocytes," *Blood* 81, no. 6 (March 15, 1993): 1540-48.
13. D. M. Bitner et al., "Enhanced Tumor Imaging with Pokeweed Mitogen," *Nuclear Medicine and Biology* 20, no. 2 (February 1993): 203-10.
14. ACS.

Eleven: *Oxygen Therapies*

1. American Cancer Society Cancer Response System: Hydrogen Peroxide and other Hyperoxygenation Therapies, February 12, 1993.
2. C. F. Nathan et al., "Anti-Tumor Effects of Hydrogen Peroxide in Vivo, *Journal of Experimental Medicine* 154 (1981).
3. Durk Pearson and Sandy Shaw, *Life Extension,* (New York: Warner Books, 1982), 103.
4. Ed McCabe, *Oxygen Therapies,* (Morrisville, New York: Energy Publications, 1988), 74-75.
5. Pearson, 803.
6. McCabe, 101.
7. P. Aubourg, "L'Ozone medical: Production, Posologie, Modes d'applications cliniques," *Bull Med Soc,* Med Paris 52 (1938), 745-49.
8. J. Sweet et al., "Ozone Selectively Inhibits Growth of Human Cancer Cells," *Science* 209 (1980): 931-33.
9. K. S. Zanker, "In Vitro Synergistic Activity of 5-Fluorouracil with Low-Dose Ozone Against a Chemoresistant Tumor Cell Line and Fresh Human Cells," *International Journal of Experimental and Clinical Chemotherapy* 36 (1990).
10. V. Bocci, "Ozonization of Blood for the Therapy of Viral Diseases and Immunodeficiencies. A Hypothesis," *Medical Hypotheses* 39, no. 1 (September 1992): 30-4.
11. Ibid.

12. ACS.
13. V. Ozmen, "Irrigation of the Abdominal Cavity in the Treatment of Experimentally Induced Microbial Peritonitis: Efficacy of Ozonated Saline," *American Surgeon* 59, no. 5 (May 1993): 297-303.
14. R. Shiratori et al., "Can Ozone Administration Activate the Tissue Metabolism?," *Masui* (Japan) 42, no. 1 (January 1993): 2-6.
15. J. Sroczynski, "Clinical Assessment of Treatment Results for Atherosclerotic Ischemia of the Lower Extremities with Intraarterial Ozone Injections," *Pol Tyg Lek* (Poland) 47, no. 42-43 (October 19-26, 1992): 964-66.
16. A. Gierek-Lapinska, "Preliminary Report on Using General Ozone Therapy in Diseases of the Posterior Segment of the Eye," *Klin Oczna* (Poland) 94, no. 5-6 (May/June 1992): 139-40.
17. F. J. Kelly and S. Birch, "Ozone Exposure Inhibits Cardiac Protein Synthesis in the Mouse," *Free Radic Biol Med* 14, no. 4 (April 1993): 443-46.
18. H. Witschi et al., "Modulation of N-nitrosodiethylamine-Induced Hamster Lung Tumors by Ozone," *Toxicology* 77, no. 1-2 (January 29, 1993): 193-202.

Twelve: *Iscador*

1. P. Heusser, "Health and Illness from an Anthroposophical Viewpoint," Lecture at the Summer Academy. Reported in *Schweiz Rundsch Med Praxis*, (Switzerland) 82, no. 1 (May 25, 1993): 629-32.
2. S. Bruseth and A. Enge, "Mistletoe in the Treatment of Cancer," *Tidsskr Nor Laegeferon*, (Norway) 113, no. 9 (March 30, 1993): 1058-60.
3. American Cancer Society Cancer Response System: Iscador, July 1, 1991.
4. Ibid.
5. R. Houston, *Repression and Reform in the Evaluation of Alternative Cancer Therapies*, (Washington, D.C.: Project Cure, 1989).
6. A. V. Timoshenko and H. J. Gabius, "Efficient Induction of Superoxide Release from Human Neutrophils by the Galactoside-specific Lectin from *Viscum album*," *Biol Chem* (Germany) 374, no. 4 (April 1993): 237-43.
7. G. Kuttan and R. Kuttan, "Reduction of Leukopenia in mice by "Viscum album" [mistletoe] Administration During Radiation and Chemotherapy," *Tumori* (Italy) 79, no. 1 (February 28, 1993): 74-6.
8. Ibid.
9. V. Bocci, "Mistletoe Lectins as Cytokine Inducers and Immunoadjuvants in Tumor Therapy. A Review," *J Biol Regul Homeost Agents* 7, no. 1 (January-March 1993): 1-6.
10. S. Brusseth.

Thirteen: *Live Cell Therapy*

1. American Cancer Society Cancer Response System: Fresh Cell Therapy, December 18, 1992.
2. Paul Niehans, *Introduction to Cellular Therapy*, (New York: Pageant Books, 1960).
3. American Cancer Society.
4. Ibid.
5. Guillemin and Rosenberg, *Endocrinology* 57 (1956): 599-607.
6. Wolfram Kuhnau, M.D., *Live-Cell Therapy: Xenotransplants*, San Ysidro, California: Self-published monograph, 1983, p. 66.

7. A. Kment, "The Objective Demonstration of the revitalization effect after cell implantations," in F. Schmid and J. Stein, *Cell Research and Cellular Therapy.* Switzerland: Ott Publishers, 1967.
8. H. Hoepke, "Cellular Therapy in Tumors," in F. Schmid and J. Stein, *Cell Research and Cellular Therapy.* Switzerland: Ott Publishers.
9. Kuhnau, Personal communication, January 18, 1993.
10. Kuhnau, *Live-Cell Therapy,* p. 110.
11. Kuhnau, Personal communication.
12. American Cancer Society.
13. Kuhnau.
14. American Cancer Society.

Fourteen: *DMSO*

1. G. Moore, *Lancet* 1 (June 5, 1976): 1238.
2. E. J. Tucker et al., *International Surgery,* 49, no. 6 (June 1968): 516.
3. American Cancer Society Cancer Response System: Dimethyl Sulfoxide, December 18, 1992.
4. ACS.
5. *Physicians' Desk Reference.* (New Jersey: Medical Economics Company, 1990) p. 1743.
6. R. Pommier et al., "Cytotoxicity of DMSO and Antineoplastic Combinations Against Human Tumors," *American Journal of Surgery* 155 (1988).
7. A. S. Salim, "Scavengers of Oxygen-derived Free Radicals Prolong Survival in Advanced Colonic Cancer. A New Approach," *Tumor Biology* 14, no. 1 (1993): 9-17.
8. *Physicians' Desk Reference,* p. 1743.

Fifteen: *Macrobiotics*

1. Michio Kushi, *The Cancer Prevention Diet,* (New York: St. Martin's Press, 1993), 133.
2. *Cancer Free,* Compiled by the East West Foundation. (New York: Japan Publications, 1991), 239.
3. T. Hirayama, "Relationship of Soybean Paste Soup Intake to Gastric Cancer Risk," *Journal of Nutrition and Cancer,* 3 (1982): 223-33.
4. J. Teas et al., "Dietary Seaweed and Mammary Carcinogenesis in Rats," *Cancer Research* 44 (1984): 2758-61.
5. I. Yamamoto et al., "Antitumor Effects of Seaweeds. I. Antitumor Effect of Extracts from Sargassum and Laminaria," *Jpn J Exp Med* 44 (1974): 543-46.
6. Vivian Newbold, "Remission of Advanced Malignant Disease: A Review of Cases with a Possible Dietary Factor," in *Cancer Free,* 236.
7. Ibid., 241-248.
8. Ibid., 248-249.
9. "Summary of a Retrospective Study of Diet and Cancer of the Pancreas," Tulane School of Public Health and Tropical Medicine, Dept. of Nutrition, 1984/1985.
10. Ibid.
11. American Cancer Society Cancer Response System: *Macrobiotics for the Treatment of Cancer,* December 12, 1992.
12. Anthony Sattilaro, M.D., *Recalled By Life.* (New York: Avon Books, 1982).
13. American Cancer Society, *Dubious Cancer Treatment,* 1991, 87.

14. American Cancer Society Cancer Response System.
15. Newbold, 250.
16. D. Miller, "Vitamin B-12 Status in a Macrobiotic Community," *American Journal of Clinical Nutrition*, no. 53 (1991).
17. American Cancer Society Cancer Response System.
18. Harriet Fels, "Testing the Macrobiotic Miracle," *The Gazette*, Montreal, Canada, (November 20, 1987).
19. Kushi, 71.

Sixteen: *Vitamins, Minerals, and Enzyme Preparations*

1. N. Wald et al., "Low Serum Vitamin A and Subsequent Risk of Cancer," *Lancet*, (October 18, 1980): 813.
2. E. W. Chu, "An Inhibitory Effect of Vitamin A in the Induction of Tumors of Forestomach and Cervix in the Syrian Hamster by Carcinogenic Polycyclic Compounds," *Cancer Research*, 10 (1965): 884.
3. M. H. Cohen, "Enhancement of Antitumor Effect of Alkylated Agents by Vitamin A," *Proceedings of the American Association for Cancer Research* (1969): 140.
4. W. Bollag, "Vitamin A and Retinoids," *Lancet* (April 16, 1983): 860.
5. P. M. Newberne, "Nutrition and Cancer: A Review With Emphasis on the Role of Vitamins C, E and Selenium," *Nutrition and Cancer* 5 (1983): 107-119.
6. C. Ip, "Attenuation of the Anticarcinogenic Action of Selenium by Vitamin E Deficiency," *Cancer Letters* 25 (1985): 325-31.
7. Robert Houston, *Repression and Reform In The Evaluation of Alternative Cancer Therapies*, (Washington, D.C.: Project Cure, 1989), 30-34.
8. H. Satoh, "Antitumor Activity of New Organogermanium Compound, GE-132," *Gan To Kagaku Ryoho* (Japan) no. 6, (1979).
9. N. Kumano et al., "Antitumor Effect of the Organogermanium Compound Ge-132 on the Lewis Lung Carcinoma (3LL) in C57BL/B6 Mice," *Tohoku J Exp Med*. (Japan) 146, (1985).
10. Senator Edward Long, "Is the FDA Hamstringing Cancer Research?," Speech, *Congressional Record* vol. 112, part 19, October 5, 1966.
11. Karl Ransberger, "Vitamin A and Proteolytic Enzymes in Cancer Chemotherapy," International Congress, Athens, 1973.
12. *Lancet* no. 7364 (October 17, 1964): 832.
13. C. J. Michet, *Congressional Record*, vol. 112 (October 14, 1966): 26913.
14. A. Rios et al., "Immunospecific Regression of Various Syngeneic Mouse Tumors in Response to Neuraminidase-treated Tumor Cells," *Journal of the National Cancer Institute* 51 (1973): 637.

Seventeen: *Metabolic Cancer Therapy*

1. H. Manner et al., "Amygdalin, Vitamin A and Enzymes Induced Regression of Murine Mammary Adenocarcinomas," *Journal of Manipulative and Physiological Therapeutics* 1, no. 4 (December 1978).
2. B. Wilson, "Dubious Degrees and Spurious Science," in *Dubious Cancer Treatment*, American Cancer Society, 1991, 49.
3. Ibid., 48.
4. J. Fink, *Third Opinion*. (New York: Avery Publishing Group, 1991), 25.
5. Geronimo Rubio, M.D., Personal communication, November 19, 1993.

6. Ibid.
7. Barrie Cassileth, "Historical Trends and Patient Characteristics," in *Dubious Cancer Treatment,* 29-30.

Eighteen: *Adjuvant Vaccine Therapies*

1. B. A. Waisbren et al., "Whole Cell Heat Killed Gram-Negative Bacilli Vaccine," *Wisconsin Medical Journal* 73 (1975): 42-5.
2. H. F. Oettgen et al., "Effects of Dialyzable Transfer Factor in Patients with Breast Cancer," *Proceedings of the National Academy of Sciences,* 71 (1974): 2319-23.
3. The Waisbren Clinic, 1993.
4. B. A. Waisbren, "Observations on the Combined Systemic Administration of Mixed Bacterial Vaccine, BCG, Transfer Factor and Lymphoblastoid Lymphocytes to Patients with Cancer, 1974-1985," *Journal of Biological Response Modifiers* 6 (1987): 1-19.
5. Ibid.
6. Ibid.
7. B. A. Waisbren, Personal communication, December 6, 1993.

Nineteen: *What You Need to Know About Choosing an Alternative Cancer Therapy*

1. Bernice Wallen, *I Beat Cancer,* New York: Contemporary Books, 1978.
2. H. L. Newbold, *Vitamin C Against Cancer,* (New York: Stein & Day Publishers, 1979), 321.
3. Ibid., 322.
4. B. A. Waisbren, "Observations on the Combined Systemic Administration of Mixed Bacterial Vaccine, BCG, Transfer Factor, and Lymphoblastoid Lymphocytes to Patients with Cancer," *Journal of Biological Response Modifiers* 6 (1987): 1-19.
5. American Cancer Society, *Dubious Cancer Treatment,* 1991, 4.
6. *Ca-A Cancer Journal for Clinicians* 41, no. 1 (January-February 1991): 20-35.
7. B. O'Reagan. *Healing, Remission and Miracle Cures,* Special report, Washington Committee of the Institute of Noetic Sciences, American University, December 5, 1986.

Glossary

Abscisic Acid: A chemical related to vitamin A which regulates the growth of plants and, some believe, the growth of tumors in people.

Accutane: A synthetic drug chemically related to vitamin A which is used to treat acne and also being experimentally used against certain forms of cancer.

Allopathy: The form of medicine most commonly practiced in the West, whereby diseases are treated with medications designed to produce effects opposite to those caused by the disease.

Amygdalin: A sugar derivative found in hundreds of plants, kernels, and seeds. Amygdalin is the chemical from which Laetrile is made and it can, under certain conditions, break down into a number of substances, including hydrogen cyanide.

Anaerobic: The ability of growing or reproducing in an environment without air or oxygen.

Antibodies: Immune-system cells that neutralize the effects of infectious organisms.

Antiemetic: A drug that prevents or controls nausea and vomiting.

Antigen: The protein found on the surfaces of bacteria, viruses, and other organisms which the immune system recognizes as "foreign" and which triggers the immune system to make antibodies.

Antioxidant: A chemical or nutrient that counteracts the oxidation of fats, oils, and other substances in the body; when oxidation occurs, free radicals form and these are known to attack and cause abnormal changes in healthy tissues leading to heart disease, aging, and cancer (see also "Free radical").

Ascorbic Acid: Vitamin C.

Assay: A test used to determine the potency of a drug or the amount of a specific chemical in a mixture.

Autogenous vaccine: A vaccine made from cultures of a patient's own bacteria or body fluids.

Autohemotherapy: The process in which blood is drawn, mixed with oxygen and ozone, then reintroduced into the body.

Bacterium: A small, single-celled microorganism having either a rod, sphere, or spiral shape and which reproduces by simple division. Some bacteria are pathogenic (disease-causing) and others are actually beneficial, such as in the process of fermentation or the breakdown of key nutrients in the intestines. Bacteria are generally larger than viruses.

B-cell: A type of white blood cell made in the bone marrow (hence the name "B" cell). B-cells are responsible for the production of disease-fighting antibodies.

BCG: (Bacillus, Calmette-Guérin) a type of vaccine made from *Mycobacterium bovis,* a tuberculosis-causing organism found in cattle and used as an immunizing agent against human tuberculosis.

Beta carotene: A substance found in brightly colored plants such as carrots, which is converted into vitamin A in the body. Beta carotene has been found to play a crucial role in the prevention and possible treatment of cancer.

Beta glucosidase: An enzyme which some scientists claim exists in higher concentration in cancer tissues. Beta glucosidase is believed to split the two sugar molecules normally joined together in the drug Laetrile so that cyanide is released, thereby killing cancer cells.

Cachexia: The devastating wasting and malnutrition syndrome that affects cancer patients—often in the advanced stages of disease.

Cell-mediated immunity: Immune-system activity in which white blood cells suppress harmful organisms through the influence of T-cells.

Chelation: The process whereby certain poisonous metals such as lead are bonded with a chemical agent and removed from the body. Some physicians believe that chelating agents can also bind with and remove atherosclerotic plaques from the arteries.

Clinical trial: A controlled study usually involving several groups of patients for the purpose of screening a particular drug or disease treatment. Clinical trials are designed to eliminate, as much as possible, any biasing factors which may prejudice the outcome and interpretation of the study results.

Control group: A group of people in a clinical trial used as a standard for comparison with the group of people actually being tested or evaluated.

Cytokines: Powerful substances produced by the body to help stimulate immunity.

Detoxification: In metabolic medicine, a purging process by which toxic materials in the body are said to be eliminated. Detoxification is believed to occur through the organs of excretion, respiration, and by way of the skin. Some holistic doctors use methods such as fasting, enemas, and diet to effect detoxification.

Differentiation: Process of organization by which healthy cells and tissues become specialized in order to perform various functions. A lack of differentiation is what defines the cancer cell's abnormality and destructiveness.

Double-blind study: A clinical study in which neither the investigator nor the patient knows who is receiving the drug or treatment being evaluated and who is receiving a fake substance known as a placebo. Only after the study is concluded are these factors revealed. The double-blind is performed so that possible biases (for example, unconscious cues or gestures) are not passed from the investigator to the patient, thus shaping or influencing the patient's responses.

Electrolyte: A substance found in bodily fluids that conducts an electric current. Electrolytes (calcium, magnesium, sodium, and potassium, for example) must exist in a state of balance with each other for health to be maintained; imbalances can result in a number of problems, including heart rhythm irregularities. Electrolyte disturbances often result from severe diarrhea, kidney problems, and malnutrition.

Epidemiology: The branch of medicine that investigates the cause, frequency, and control of a disease in a given population.

Fermentation: The theoretical process by which cancer cells derive energy. According to this theory, cancer cells do not breathe in oxygen and give off carbon dioxide the way normal cells do; instead, they break down or *ferment* blood sugars in the absence of oxygen.

Five-year survival: The time frame which, in the absence of any recurrence of a patient's cancer, constitutes a cure.

Free radical: An unstable atom or molecule that forms under a number of conditions such as when fatty acids are oxidized (i.e., react with oxygen). Free radicals are short-lived, reactive molecules that can attack healthy tissue and contribute to aging, heart disease and cancer (see also "Antioxidant").

Gram: A basic unit of measurement which is approximately $1/28$ of an ounce. One gram equals 1,000 milligrams.

HCG: (Human chorionic gonadotropin), a pregnancy hormone that supports fetal growth and is believed to play a crucial role in protecting the developing embryo from attack by the immune system. Some researchers think that HCG is also utilized by cancer cells as a means of avoiding immune-system attack.

Interleukins: Protein factors that stimulate the immune system and are involved in the activation of "T" and other disease-fighting cells. Interleukins also act as messengers between immune-system cells (see also "Interleukin-2").

Interleukin-2: An interleukin-based drug that is highly toxic and has been tried with limited success against several forms of cancer (see also "Interleukins").

Koch's postulates: A set of laws which prove the connection between a causative agent such as a bacterium and a specific disease.

Lectins: Plant proteins that stimulate the production of white blood cells.

Leucovorin rescue: Medical technique in which a potentially lethal dose of a folic-acid–inhibiting cancer drug is administered and then neutralized by the drug leucovorin before fatal complications set in.

Leukopenia: An abnormal decrease in the number of white blood cells. Leukopenia often results from a toxic reaction to cancer drugs and radiation exposure.

Lymphoblastoid Lymphocytes: Living white blood cells derived from patients under the stress of infection. These cells help the immune system reject cancer cells the way donor organs are rejected by transplant recipients.

Lymphoma: A type of cancer which affects tissues of the lymphatic system. Hodgkin's disease and lymphatic leukemia are two types of lymphomas.

Marker: (see "Antigen").

Megadose: An amount or dose of a substance which exceeds the usual recommended dosage by hundreds or thousands of times. Megadose usually applies to the application of vitamins, minerals, and other nutrients in medical treatment.

Melanoma: A melanin-derived tumor which affects the skin and is sometimes malignant.

Mesothelioma: A rare type of cancer that affects the lining of the lungs and is often the result of exposure to asbestos. Mesothelioma generally has a very poor prognosis.

Metabolic medicine: An eclectic approach to cancer treatment which focuses on reversing the underlying causes of cancer by restoring healthy immunity, "detoxifying" the body, and potentiating the patient's natural tumor-fighting abilities. Metabolic physicians generally employ both nondrug and drug approaches to treatment.

Mitogen: A substance that induces and regulates cell division.

Mixed Bacterial Vaccine (MBV): A type of vaccine made from different strains or species of bacteria, including those infecting burn patients. MBV is believed to stimulate immunity and the production of cancer-killing *tumor necrosis factor.*

Necrosis: The death of cells or tissues which results from injury, disease, or inadequate blood supply.

Neuraminidase: A virus-derived enzyme which causes some cancer cells to become more susceptible to destruction via the immune system. Neuraminidase is believed to neutralize HCG—the growth hormone which, some evidence suggests, can shield both cancer cells and the human fetus from the immune system (see also "HCG").

Objective stabilization: In cancer treatment, the measurable cessation of cancer growth.

Observed survival: The actual or true rate of people surviving cancer. In 1990, the observed survival rate was 40 percent.

Orthomolecular: The branch of medicine that treats and prevents disease by administering the correct amounts of nutrients. Based on individual requirements, the doses of nutrients given can exceed hundreds of times the recommended daily allowances.

Peer review: The scrutiny given a scientific paper or medical claim by independent reviewers.

Peptides: Two or more amino acids linked together by a peptide bond.

Placebo: An inert substance having no medicinal value. Placebos are used in double-blind studies as a means of objectively assessing the effect of the real medicine being evaluated.

Positive bias: A factor which favorably influences the health of a cancer patient, but falsely bolsters the actual worth of the treatment in question—thus biasing the results.

Prospective trial: A clinically controlled study which investigates and follows the effects of a medical treatment through to its natural conclusion. In a prospective trial, the end results are not known until the trial's completion.

Proteolytic: The breaking down of proteins by enzymes.

Relative survival: The potential cancer cure rate based on numerical projections—not actual mortality data. The relative survival estimate of 50 percent is often used to depict the true cure rate (see also "observed survival").

Retrospective trial: A study which compares patients receiving a drug or medical treatment with other nonparticipating patients who have already experienced the disease or condition being treated.

Rhodanese: An enzyme believed to neutralize the effects of cyanide. Laetrile proponents claim that normal cells have higher concentrations of this enzyme than cancer cells and are thus selectively protected from cyanide-releasing drugs such as Laetrile.

Scavenger: Any substance which counteracts the dangerous effects of free radicals.

Sodium ascorbate: The sodium or salt version of ascorbic acid (vitamin C).

Spontaneous remission: The remission of cancer not due to any known treatment or cause. Spontaneous remissions are extremely rare.

Statistical artifact: The favorable alteration of a disease based on historical factors and not necessarily medical ones. For example, while the death rate from stomach cancer has declined, so has the incidence of the disease—irrespective of any advances in medical technology.

Superoxide dismutase (SOD): An enzyme that reacts with free radicals and converts them to less dangerous molecules. SOD is believed to prevent possible free-radical damage associated with the medical use of hydrogen peroxide.

T-cell: Immune system cells derived from the *thymus* gland (hence the name "T" cell) which are involved in cell-mediated immunity.

Testimonial: A personal claim of cure or remission not necessarily based on scientific fact or documentation.

Titer: The amount of antibodies reacting to a specific infection in a measured unit of serum.

Transfer Factor: Immune-system cells taken from healthy donors and given to cancer patients. Transfer factor transfers the disease recognition/destruction abilities of the donor cells to the immune-system cells of the patient receiving the factor.

Tumor Factor: A protein which triggers cells to become cancerous.

Tumor Necrosis Factor (TNF): A protein originally made from the immune systems of animals exposed to bacterial proteins. When certain tumors are exposed to TNF, they necrose—i.e., shrivel up and die. TNF is potentially toxic and has not shown universally successful effects against human cancers.

Virus: An extremely minute particle that can only reproduce by injecting its genetic materials into a separate, living cell and using that cell's nucleic acid to make carbon copies of itself. Newly formed viruses burst out of their host cell and go on to infect and parasitize other cells. Viruses are so minute that they generally pass through special laboratory filters which can trap all but the smallest organisms (see also "Bacteria").

Weasel words: Words or phrases that are misleading and deceptive. Unethical medical practitioners sometimes use weasel words to sell a product or convince patients that a treatment is effective even though the reverse is true.

Suggested Reading

I Beat Cancer, Bernice Wallen. Contemporary Books, 1978. (One patient's account of investigating and utilizing an alternative cancer therapy despite much opposition.)

The Conquest of Cancer, Virginia Livingston-Wheeler. New York: Franklin Watts, 1984.

The Cancer Industry, Ralph Moss. New York: Paragon House, 1989. (An indispensable overview of the politics and economic forces long resisting alternative cancer therapies.)

Third Opinion, John M. Fink. Second Edition. Garden City: Avery Publishing Group, 1992. (A useful directory of alternative cancer therapies.)

Vitamin C Against Cancer, H. L. Newbold, M.D. New York: Stein & Day, 1979.

Repression and Reform in the Evaluation of Alternative Cancer Therapies, Robert G. Houston. Project Cure: Washington, 1989.

The Cancer Survivors. Judith Glassman. New York: Dial Press, 1983.

World Without Cancer, Part Two, Edward Griffin. California: American Media, 1980 (important reading describing how political and economic forces have shaped medical research and priorities.)

Vitamins Against Cancer, Kedar N. Prasad. Nutrition Publishing House, Inc., 1989.

Vitamin C and Cancer. Medicine or Politics? Evelleen Richards. New York: St. Martin's Press, 1991.

Index

M

MacDonald, Ian, 101
Macrobiotics, 147–152, 179, 180
Magnesium, 153
Malignant melanoma, 149, 168
Manner cocktail, 161
Manner, Harold, 161, 162, 164, 174
Margaret Mead Film Festival, 128
Martin, Daniel S., 103
Maugham, Somerset, 139
Mayo Clinic, 66, 82, 86, 91, 92, 95–96, 105
Mazet, George, 28
McCarty, Mark, 99
McGrady, Patrick, 155
Medical fraud, 178
Mehl, John W., 101
Mercury astronaut program, 60
Mesothelioma, 73
Metabolic Research Foundation, 163
Metabolic therapy, 161–165
Methotrexate, 13
Middlesex Hospital, 24
Miley, George, 37, 41, 42
Miller, Mildred, 145
Miso soup, 148
Mistletoe, 135, 137
Mistletoe lectin, 137
Mitogens, 127
Mixed Bacterial Vaccine (MBV), 26, 166, 167
Moertel, Charles, 91–93, 105
Molinari, Guy, 70, 73, 74, 77
Molybdenum, 153
Montpellier Médecine, 28
Morrone, John, 101
Moss, Ralph, 103, 106, 119
Motion therapy, 136
Music therapy, 136
Mycoplasma, 167

N

National Academy of Sciences, 145
National Advisory Cancer Council, 31
National Cancer Act, 3
National Cancer Center (Tokyo), 115

National Cancer Institute (NCI), 4, 8, 43, 55, 65, 66, 67, 69, 75, 76, 77, 90, 91, 104, 105, 106, 110, 115–119, 157, 170
National Health Fraud Conference, 77
National Institutes of Health (NIH), 94, 169, 182
Nattenberg, Maurice, 25
Nature, 57
Nausea, 13, 18
Nauts, Helen Coley, 26
Naval Medical Research Institute, 31
Navarro, Madrazo, 142
Navarro, Manuel, 101, 102
Needle biopsy, 9
Neihans, Paul, 139, 140
Nelson, Mildred, 126
Nerve inflammation, 141
Neuraminidase, 157
Newbold, H. L., 171, 172
Newbold, Vivian, 149, 150
New England Journal of Medicine (NEJM), 4, 8, 57, 79, 91, 93, 94, 105
New Jersey Freedom of Choice Committee, 105
New Scientist, 87
Newton, Issac, 87
New York Times, 57
New York University School of Medicine, 48
Ninth International Symposium on Future Trends in Chemotherapy, 114
Nocardia asteroides, 81
Non-specific vaccine, 163
Nori, 148
Northwestern University, 163
Null, Gary, 78
Nuremberg trials, 31
Nutrition and Cancer, 60

O

Observed survival rate, 5, 7
Obstructive pulmonary disease, 13
Ochoa, Manuel, 62
Office of Alternative Medicine, 182

ABOUT THE AUTHOR

Ron Falcone spent the last eight years interviewing medical professionals and researching alternative cancer therapies for this book. He
is a free-lance journalist based in Central Florida. His articles have
appeared in publications such as *Your Health, Florida Magazine,* and
Woman's Day. He lives in Sanford, Florida, with his wife and their
three children.